6/20/01

To Scott

With best wishes

Bill Jacott

Champions *of* Quality
in Health Care

Champions *of* Quality
in Health Care

A History of the Joint

Commission on Accreditation

of Healthcare Organizations

Carl M. Brauer

Greenwich Publishing Group, Inc.
Lyme, Connecticut

The mission of the Joint Commission on Accreditation of Healthcare Organizations is to continuously improve the safety and quality of the care provided to the public through the provision of health care accreditation and related services that support performance improvement in health care organizations.

ABOUT THE AUTHOR

Carl M. Brauer, a freelance historian and biographer, lives and works in Belmont, Massachusetts. He has written or edited many books, oral histories, memoirs, and articles, including several on health care institutions and practitioners. Brauer received his Ph.D. in history from Harvard University in 1973. Until 1989 he taught and did research at leading universities, including the University of Virginia and Harvard University.

PHOTO CREDITS

Page 14 courtesy of the American College of Surgeons
Page 20 courtesy of the American College of Surgeons
Page 23 courtesy of the American College of Surgeons
    and the American Hospital Association
Page 25 courtesy of the American College of Surgeons
Page 27 courtesy of the American College of Surgeons
    and the American Hospital Association
Page 28 courtesy of the American College of Surgeons
Page 29 courtesy of the American College of Surgeons
Page 33 courtesy of the American Hospital Association
Page 35 courtesy of the American Hospital Association
Page 40 courtesy of the American Hospital Association
Page 50 courtesy of Chicago Historical Society
Page 60 courtesy of the American Hospital Association
Pages 64 and 65 courtesy of © G. E. Kidder Smith/CORBIS
Pages 125 and 130 photographed by Diane Alexander White
All other images courtesy of the Joint Commission on Accreditation of Healthcare Organizations

Produced and published by Greenwich Publishing Group, Inc., Lyme, Connecticut

Design by Dutton & Sherman Design

Library of Congress Catalog Card Number: 00-112092

ISBN: 0-944641-45-8

First Printing: January 2001

Contents

Preface

The Joint Commission on Accreditation of Healthcare Organizations commissioned this history and fully cooperated in its preparation. Dennis S. O'Leary, the Joint Commission's president, encouraged me to write a truthful account and not to gloss over its "checkered history." His attitude is very much in keeping with the Joint Commission's purpose of shining a light into the dark corners of an organization so that problems may be better addressed.

I have tried to present a balanced history of the Joint Commission but make no attempt to predict its future. I had access to all of the Joint Commission's board minutes and publications, as well as to internal records and reports that I requested. I interviewed more than 50 current and former staff and board members in addition to knowledgeable observers and outsiders. Everyone was open and helpful. Several individuals dug into their own files and loaned me interesting documents. I also benefited from informal conversations with friends and acquaintances in the health care field.

One thing in particular has come through very strongly in the course of my research: those involved in the Joint Commission's work, whether staff or board members, all believe deeply in its mission. At different times, people connected to the Joint

Commission have wondered and worried about its continued relevance, effectiveness, or responsiveness, but there never has been any doubt about its central purpose. Everyone believes that assuring high quality health care is a vitally important objective, ultimately involving life and death. Indeed, the high stakes help explain why debate surrounding the Joint Commission's activities can at times become emotional.

This book gives an overview of the Joint Commission's history, focusing on major developments in policy, personnel, and organization. I have tried to include enough interesting particulars and anecdotes to make the story lively and human without becoming bogged down in details. I have tried to focus on the forest, not the trees. The particular woods occupied by the Joint Commission are thick, the paper from those woods even thicker. I was mindful of broader developments and trends in health care and society, which in many ways were reflected in what the Joint Commission was doing or not doing at any particular time. But again my focus was on the Joint Commission itself, not on its external environment.

Carl M. Brauer
December 2000

Introduction

The overarching purpose of the Joint Commission on Accreditation of Healthcare Organizations is to improve the safety and quality of health care provided to the public in organized delivery settings. The Joint Commission sets standards for, evaluates, and accredits nearly 20,000 health care organizations and programs in the United States. These include over 11,000 of the nation's hospitals and home health agencies and more than 8,000 other organizations, including ambulatory care services, behavioral health programs, clinical laboratories, health care networks, and long-term care organizations. Widely recognized as the world's preeminent accrediting body in the health field, the Joint Commission also provides educational and consulting services to professionals, organizations, and agencies in the United States and around the globe.

The organization was founded as the Joint Commission on Accreditation of Hospitals in 1951 by a collaboration of four leading provider organizations: the American College of Surgeons (ACS), the American Hospital Association (AHA), the American Medical Association (AMA), and the American College of Physicians (ACP). In fact, the Joint Commission was created to take over the work of a hospital standardization program initiated by the ACS in 1918. Since that time, the ACS's standardiza-tion program had significantly advanced the quality of care by establishing standards and by inspecting and certifying hospitals that met them. But the need for the program had outgrown its funding mechanism. Recognizing the importance of the program, the four founding organizations agreed to work together in a new entity dedicated to the purpose of hospital accreditation.

The Joint Commission's 50th anniversary is an opportunity to look back and take stock of where it has been and what it has accomplished. As an organization, it has undergone great change, but there have also been some distinct continuities. When the Joint Commission began to operate in 1952, it had a professional staff of two and an annual budget of $70,000, a sum which came entirely from dues paid by its corporate members, the organizations which founded it. The vast majority of its surveyors, the professionals who went out into the field to inspect and accredit hospitals, also came from these member organizations. In 2000, the Joint Commission had a headquarters staff of more than 500 and employed another 650 surveyors in the field, many full-time and others part-time or intermittent. All of its surveyors were health care professionals and many of its other employees were as well. An annual budget of $127 million funded their efforts. The growth in the size and capabilities of the Joint Commission's professional staff manifests one obvious change over these 50 years.

To be sure, the Joint Commission's growth has largely reflected the overall growth in the American health care industry, where total annual expenditures were recently estimated to be about $1.2 trillion. In strictly dollar terms, the Joint Commission budget represents about 0.0001 percent of health care related spending in the United States. It is fair to say that the Joint Commission's impact exceeds its relatively diminutive size. The standards it establishes ripple through the entire health care sector. However, the actual effects of the Joint Commission's standards and activities have never received careful documentation or systematic measurement. It would be a daunting task to differentiate what the Joint Commission did from other developments that were taking place simultaneously and might have proceeded in any event.

The Joint Commission and its antecedent hospital certification program are distinctly American-type institutions in that they are voluntary, private solutions to public problems, a phenomenon described by the famed student of American politics and institutions, Frenchman Alexis de Tocqueville, after he visited the United States in the 1830s. The federal government placed great reliance on the ACS's certification program in 1946 when it enacted legislation to fund hospital construction around the country. The public

role of the Joint Commission was greatly augmented by the passage of Medicare legislation in 1965. Under this law, hospitals accredited by the Joint Commission were "deemed" to be in compliance with most of the Medicare conditions of participation and thus able to receive government reimbursement. In the view of many, the legislation effectively made the Joint Commission a quasi-government organization, opening it to greater government oversight and much more public scrutiny. Pressures toward greater disclosure and accountability have grown steadily at the Joint Commission since then. Among other things, they have led to an expansion of its board to include six public members and one at-large nurse representative. But the original corporate structure has remained, except that the American Dental Association was added as a corporate member in 1979.

The Joint Commission is the only private sector entity that is entrusted by the government with quality oversight of an industry that affects individuals' most basic right to live. Because of both its complex nature and vitally important role, the Joint Commission is often in the crossfire of criticism. It is also generally not well understood, even by its many stakeholders. Within the health care field, it is respected, revered, and admired...and it is feared, disliked, and dismissed. It is sometimes viewed as a brave pioneer and visionary leader and sometimes seen as a painfully slow and reactive bureaucracy.

Critics compare it to the "fox watching the hen house" and chastise it for being "provider-dominated and controlled." Defenders note that it performs its job better — more effectively and efficiently — than the government could precisely because it is voluntary and gets "buy-in" from those health care organizations and professionals who know it best and therefore help to set standards and measures.

At the center of the controversy is the Joint Commission's accreditation program. Although quality has always been its focus, definitions of what constitutes quality — of what the standards should be and how they are measured — have changed continuously over time. Starting in the 1980s, the Joint Commission shifted its emphasis from measuring the stated capability of health care organizations to measuring their actual performance. Interestingly, this shift marked a return to the vision of one of the Joint Commission's progenitors, Ernest Amory Codman, who in the early years of the twentieth century urged doctors and hospitals to develop systems of measuring "end results." Following the lead of other industries, the Joint Commission began to promote "continuous quality improvement" and began to emphasize a more systems-oriented approach to assuring quality and safety.

Although the Joint Commission has sometimes been seen by its immediate customers as a distant Mount Olympus handing down edicts from on high, its very composition has always meant that standards have been set through a process of negotiation, give-and-take, and sometimes contentious debate among health care professionals, the organizations that represent them, and those having strong interests in the influence and outcomes of the accreditation process. The debate involves both professional values and a variety of firmly held beliefs and — usually under the surface — money, power, and self-interest as well.

Standard setting has never been a simple process, and it has only become more complex as new technologies and new ways of delivering care have come on line. Scientific, technological, and methodological developments have been accompanied by increased specialization, sub-specialization, and a proliferation of new professional organizations, continuously complicating the negotiation process. Despite the complexity of this process — or perhaps as a result of it — the quality standards the Joint Commission establishes become widely accepted in the field, if they had not been accepted there before. And whatever flaws remain in the accreditation process, this steady push toward uniformity and improved quality of services and treatment allows health care professionals to perform their work to a superior standard wherever they happen to be.

From Standardization to the Creation of the Joint Commission

ORIGINS OF STANDARDIZATION

Standardization of hospitals grew out of a rich soil of developments in science, medicine, and society. In the last third of the nineteenth century, scientists began to uncover the infectious basis of deadly diseases, including anthrax, gonorrhea, malaria, pneumonia, typhoid fever, tetanus, influenza, bubonic plague, and dysentery. Discoveries about such diseases created optimism about scientific medicine, where clear causes and effects could be observed and proven. At the end of the nineteenth century and the beginning of the twentieth century, advances in anesthesia and antisepsis and the diagnostic application of x-rays expanded surgery's capability, promise, and safety.

In these same years, medicine underwent significant reform as a profession. The American Medical Association (AMA), established in 1847, campaigned to raise standards in medical education, medical ethics, and state licensing, while philanthropic foundations upgraded selected medical schools and associated hospitals. A key moment in professional reform was the 1910 report on medical education by Abraham Flexner of the Carnegie Foundation. One of Flexner's recommendations was that medical schools operate in association with hospitals. Prior to the adoption of this recommendation, it had been possible to graduate from medical school without ever seeing or caring for patients.

These advances gave the American public reason to invest in and support the transformation of hospitals from charitable asylums for the indigent into modern scientific institutions. New hospitals proliferated. They were started by churches and religious denominations, municipalities, counties and states, industrialists, committees of prominent citizens, ethnic and women's groups, and doctors — especially surgeons — who relied on hospitals as their workshops. Hospital births began to outnumber home births, and people began to see hospitals as places where afflictions could be cured. The growth in hos-

MEDICAL EDUCATION IN THE UNITED STATES AND CANADA

A REPORT TO
THE CARNEGIE FOUNDATION
FOR THE ADVANCEMENT OF TEACHING

BY
ABRAHAM FLEXNER

WITH AN INTRODUCTION BY
HENRY S. PRITCHETT
PRESIDENT OF THE FOUNDATION

BULLETIN NUMBER FOUR

576 FIFTH AVENUE
NEW YORK CITY

pitals constituted a prominent feature of America in the early twentieth century. Editor John Hornsby of *Modern Healthcare* estimated in 1917 that $1.445 billion was then invested in hospital land and buildings.

Simultaneously, important ideas about efficiency and standardization were emerging from other industries. Engineering, a profession at the center of a rapidly industrializing and urbanizing society, valued observation, measurement, precision, perfectibility, and results. Engineers promoted standardization as a way of increasing efficiency and reducing errors. Standardization became a popular objective in a wide range of endeavors and enterprises, leading to the establishment of the National Bureau of Standards in the U.S. Department of Commerce in 1901, which was given a broad mandate to establish and disseminate standards.

In 1895, Frederick Winslow Taylor published his first paper on scientific management, which applied rational principles to industrial processes and was aimed at optimizing efficiency. Through time and motion studies, Taylor and other engineers, including Frank and Lillian Gilbreth, studied ways in which workers could perform their tasks more efficiently and thereby increase productivity. Stopwatches and close monitoring were detested by manufacturing workers but relished by employers, who could achieve higher profits through increased productivity. Efficiency also promised to benefit consumers. In 1910, Louis D. Brandeis, the Boston lawyer and reformer who was later named to the United States Supreme Court by President Woodrow Wilson, had scientific management experts appear in the "Eastern Rate Case." These experts testified that with better management, railroads could save millions of dollars and therefore would not have to raise rates to their customers.

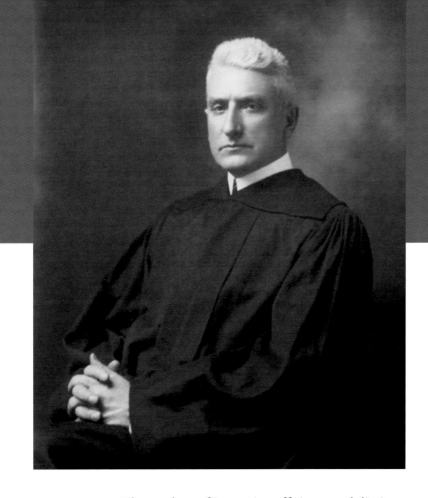

These values of increasing efficiency and diminishing errors were shared by the new generation of scientifically oriented doctors. Franklin H. Martin, an energetic Chicago surgeon, became an important leader in the medical profession as a proponent of shared knowledge. In 1905, Martin established the highly successful journal, *Surgery, Gynecology & Obstetrics*, to advance specialist knowledge. Martin realized that surgeons had to do more than read about new procedures, however — they had to observe them. So he organized the first Clinical Congress of Surgeons, which met in Chicago in 1910. It attracted 1,300 practitioners to observe in the clinics of Albert J. Ochsner, John B. Murphy, Arthur Dean Bevan, and other leading Chicago-area surgeons. Bevan and Murphy were leaders in the AMA, but it was the Clinical Congress of Surgeons, not the AMA, which offered practical postgraduate education. The AMA was busy reforming medical education and medical ethics.

Following on the success of this first Clinical Congress of Surgeons, subsequent ones were held in Philadelphia in 1911 and New York in 1912, which attracted 2,600 doctors. This enormous popularity led Martin to think about ways to restrict attendance to a manageable number. Another problem that arose in New York was the refusal of some of the better surgeons to be scheduled on the same programs with surgeons whom they regarded as their inferiors. "A crucial problem was emerging," wrote historian Rosemary Stevens, "Should the primary focus of surgical education be on upgrading the lowest common denominator to a standard of comparative safety; or should it be to create a relatively small, recognizable group of quality?" Should the focus be democratic or elitist? And who was to make this difficult decision?

At the conclusion of the New York congress, Martin proposed the formation of an American College of Surgeons modeled after the elitist Royal College of Surgeons in England, Ireland, and Scotland. Martin wanted to recognize the distinction between those who were trained surgical specialists and those who were not. He proposed a form of surgical certification beyond the medical degree and also raised the possibility of separate licensure for surgeons. John Murphy, Albert Ochsner, a prominent gynecologist from Philadelphia named Edward Martin, and other surgical leaders at the New York congress embraced these ideas. A committee, under Franklin Martin's chairmanship, was appointed to set the plan in motion.

The American College of Surgeons (ACS) was incorporated in Illinois in 1913. Four hundred and fifty surgeons from the United States and Canada attended its first meeting and were pleased to become members of this elite group. By the end of 1914, 2,700 fellows had been admitted by selection, and they proudly placed the fellowship designation, FACS, after their MDs. From the outset, the AMA was ambivalent and divided about the college, however. While some AMA leaders were prominent surgeons who joined the ACS themselves, most of the AMA's rank and file members were general practitioners whose licenses already gave them the legal right to perform surgery. They certainly did not want an elite group of surgical specialists to undercut their professional image or deny them the income they derived from performing surgery. The AMA rallied against separate licensure for surgeons, successfully holding the line at credentialing. Ironically, the AMA fully supported the Flexner report and was simultaneously waging its own elitist war on the poorer medical schools. A measure of its success was that the number of medical schools decreased from 155 in 1909 to 76 in 1930. This was

less of a reduction than Flexner had originally proposed, but it still represented a great success.

In addition to launching the ACS, the New York Clinical Congress of Surgeons in 1912 passed a resolution "that some system of standardization of hospital equipment and hospital work should be developed." Five prominent surgeons were appointed to a Hospital Standardization Committee. Ernest A. Codman of Boston was named chairman, and the other members were Walter W. Chipman of Montreal, John G. Clark of Philadelphia, Allen B. Kanavel of Chicago, and William J. Mayo of Rochester, Minnesota, who — with his brother, Charles — co-founded the Mayo Clinic. Hospital standardization was one of the stated purposes of the ACS at its inception in 1912, and the Codman committee became a standing committee of the ACS.

CODMAN AND THE END RESULT IDEA

Codman is worth examining in some detail. A descendant of Pilgrims, he was born in Boston in 1869 to a prosperous Brahmin family. Although in recent years he is often referred to as Ernest Codman, he himself almost never used his first name. According to biographer William J. Mallon, in his early life, his family and friends called him by his middle name Amory, pronounced "Emery." In his later years, he was usually known as "Cod." Codman graduated from Saint Mark's boarding school in Massachusetts, from

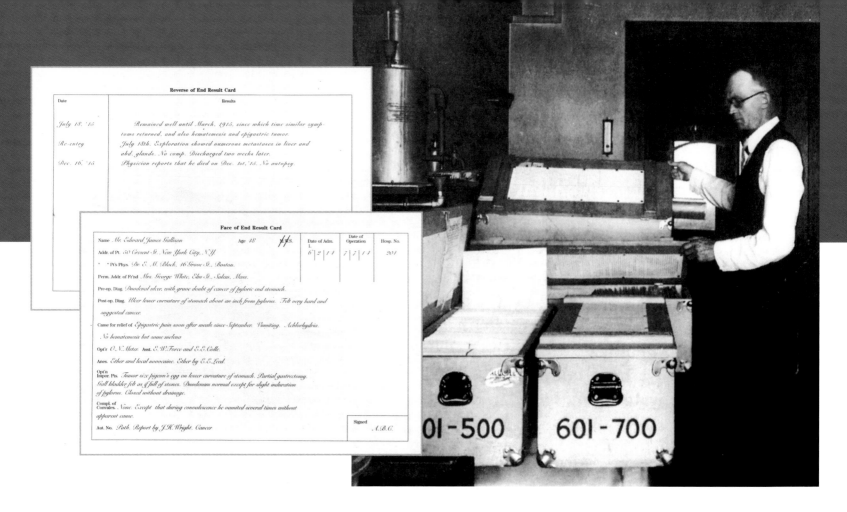

Reverse of End Result Card

Date	Results
July 18, '15	*Remained well until March, 1915, since which time similar symptoms returned, and also hematemesis and epigastric tumor.*
Re-entry	*July 18th. Exploration showed numerous metastases in liver and abd. glands. No comp. Discharged two weeks later.*
Dec. 16, '15	*Physician reports that he died on Dec. 1st, '15. No autopsy.*

Face of End Result Card

Name *Mr. Edward James Gallison* Age *18*
Addr. of Pt. *50 Crescent St. New York City, N.Y.*
Pt's Phys. *Dr. E. M. Black, 16 Grove St., Boston.*
Perm. Addr. of Fr'nd *Mrs. George White, Elm St., Salem, Mass.*
Pre-op. Diag. *Duodenal ulcer, with grave doubt of cancer of pyloric end stomach.*
Post-op. Diag. *Ulcer lesser curvature of stomach about an inch from pylorus. Felt very hard and suggested cancer.*
Cause for relief of *Epigastric pain soon after meals since September. Vomiting. Achlorhydria. No hematemesis but some melena*
Opt'r *O. N. Meter.* Asst. *E. W. Force and E. S. Colle.*
Anes. *Ether and local novocaine. Ether by E. S. Leed.*
Opt'n Impor. Pts. *Tumor size pigeon's egg on lesser curvature of stomach. Partial gastrectomy. Gall bladder felt as if full of stones. Duodenum normal except for slight induration of pylorus. Closed without drainage.*
Compl. of Convales. *None. Except that during convalescence he vomited several times without apparent cause.*
Aut. No. *Path. Report by J. H. Wright. Cancer*
Signed *A. B. C.*

Date of Adm. I. *6 | 2 | 11*
Date of Operation *7 | 7 | 11*
Hosp. No. *201*

601-500   601-700

Harvard College, and in 1895 from Harvard Medical School. Even as a young man, Codman was attracted to precision, measurement, and efficiency. An avid hunter since boyhood, he began when he was just 20 to keep a complete log of the ratio of birds shot to shells expended as a measure of hunting efficiency.

In medical school, he formed what became a life-long friendship with Harvey Cushing, who founded modern neurosurgery. While they were interning at Massachusetts General Hospital in their final year of medical school, Codman and Cushing worked on "ether charts," the first instance of monitoring a patient's anesthetic course during surgery. The charts had been suggested by Francis B. Harrington, the hospital's surgical chief, and they marked Codman's first foray into monitoring results. Codman wrote a long paper on the results but was discouraged from

publishing it because his inclusion of patient deaths could embarrass the hospital.

As a young doctor, Codman took the first x-ray in Boston and became the first radiologist (skiagrapher) at Children's Hospital. He soon left radiology, however, and was appointed an assistant surgeon at Massachusetts General Hospital. There he did pioneering work on duodenal ulcers and on shoulder injuries. It was in the latter area that he achieved his greatest fame as a surgeon. But Codman's importance exceeded any one malady or part of the anatomy.

Soon after starting his surgical practice, Codman formulated the End Result Idea, proposing that surgical patients be closely monitored after treatment to determine outcomes. Codman developed an elaborate card system for recording and reporting his own sur-

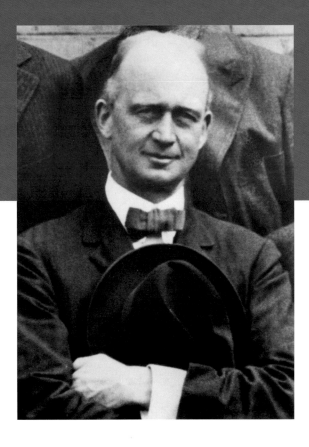

gical results, and he urged other surgeons and hospitals to do likewise. Florence Nightingale, the English founder of modern nursing during the Crimean War, had previously urged hospitals and doctors to report surgical outcomes in a standardized manner, but there is no evidence that Codman knew that she had preceded him. Codman was certainly influenced, however, by contemporary engineering ideas. Codman attended Taylor Society meetings (after Frederick Winslow Taylor) and became a friend of efficiency expert Frank Gilbreth. He was also influenced by the scientific method of experimentation as propounded by British chemist William Thompson, who was knighted as Lord Kelvin.

Initially, Codman's espousal of the End Result Idea may have been motivated in part by ambition. He chafed under the rigid seniority system at Massachusetts General Hospital, and he may have wanted to use statistics on outcomes to demonstrate his superiority to more senior surgeons there. But he became such a zealous crusader for his idea that it is hard to imagine ambition remaining a primary motive for long. In 1911, he opened a 20-bed proprietary hospital that was organized around the End Result Idea. He even offered a money-back warranty to patients, a radical proposition both then and today. For each patient, Codman maintained an end-result card, which included presenting symptoms, initial diagnosis, treatment given, in-hospital complica-

tions, discharge diagnosis, and the result a year later. Codman developed a classification method for errors and adverse outcomes, and he published his results in the hospital's report, openly documenting and reporting errors and deaths. (It should be noted that this was before the advent of medical malpractice lawsuits.) Codman gave the report to prospective patients. He also distributed it to notable hospitals around the country and encouraged them to follow his lead.

In his home precincts, however, Codman was meeting resistance and indifference, and he began to lash out at eminent local institutions and individuals. "They all knew that nobody was responsible for examining the results of treatment at hospitals, and that the reason was MONEY; in other words, that the staffs are not paid [doctors were not hospital employees; they billed patients separately for their services],

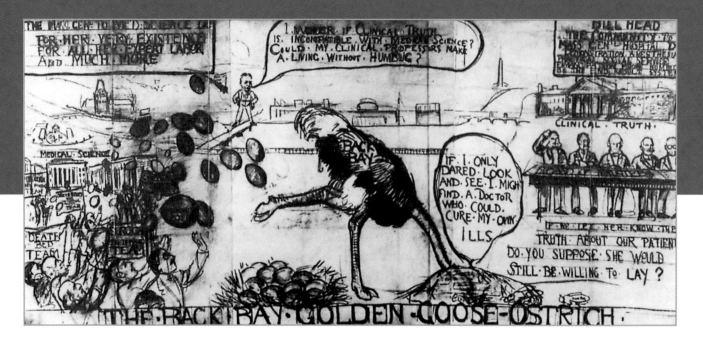

▲ *A zealous proponent of the End Result Idea, Codman sometimes stepped on people's toes. After Codman presented this satirical cartoon at a meeting of Boston surgeons in 1915, he was ostracized by the local medical establishment.*

and therefore cannot be held accountable," Codman later wrote. Codman organized and chaired a fateful meeting of the Suffolk District Medical Society held at the Boston Medical Library on January 3, 1915. The evening's subject was hospital efficiency. Among the speakers were engineer Frank Gilbreth and gynecologist Robert Dickinson, who practiced at the Women's Hospital in Brooklyn, a pioneer in the implementation of the End Result Idea.

Speaking last, Codman had Gilbreth unveil a large cartoon he had commissioned for the occasion. The cartoon depicted an ostrich, representing well-to-do Boston patients, with its head in the sand kicking out golden eggs to Back Bay physicians, who gladly accepted them. The cartoon depicted administrators of the Boston hospitals as oblivious to the results of patient care and only interested in obtaining their own golden eggs. Also seen in the cartoon were the

president of Harvard University and the dean of its medical school.

The cartoon and Codman's impolitic remarks angered and insulted many members of the audience, a number of whom walked out in disgust. The medical contretemps was reported in Boston newspapers, which was unusual at the time, and word soon filtered out to the medical profession beyond Boston. "For weeks, some of my friends did not speak to me," Codman later recounted, "and if I entered a room where other doctors gathered, the party broke up from embarrassment or changed their subject. I was asked to resign as Chairman of the local Medical Society." Even many of those who agreed with Codman's point of view were put off by his tactlessness.

Codman's career in Boston immediately suffered. Referrals to him from other doctors fell off dramatically, so that by the end of the year, the Codman Hospital was failing financially. Codman resigned from the chairmanship of the Hospital Standardization Committee. With Harvard and Massachusetts General Hospital determined to suppress him and the public not yet believing in him, Codman explained to ACS president John Finney that he could "do more by trying to make my own hospital a success than by criticizing other hospitals all over the country." In fact, Codman methodically documented the record of his own hospital in his book, *A Study in Hospital Efficiency: As Demonstrated by the Case Report of the First Five Years of a Private Hospital*, which appeared in 1918.

Codman traveled to Halifax, Nova Scotia, in December 1917 to help victims of the disastrous explosion and fire that had occurred in its harbor. He subsequently entered the army and returned to Boston in late 1919. Practically broke at that point, he threw himself back into active practice and research, taking a step back from medical reform. He converted the Codman Hospital, which had been closed in 1918, into an apartment house. He apparently reached some accommodation with Massachusetts General Hospital, because in 1925, he was given an office at the hospital. There he did studies based on the valuable Registry of Bone Sarcoma, which contained the records of failure, success, x-ray films, pathological slides, and follow-up studies of hundreds of bone cancer patients. He had initiated this registry after treating an unfortunate young man with fatal bone cancer whose wealthy father underwrote the registry's start-up costs. In 1929, Codman was appointed to Massachusetts General's consulting staff. Five years later, he privately published his magnum opus on shoulder injuries, in which he also discussed his earlier reform efforts. "The End Result Idea may not achieve fulfillment for several generations....Honors except for those I have thrust on myself are conspicuously absent in my chart, but I am able to enjoy the hypothesis that I may receive some [honors] from a more receptive generation." The prophetic Codman died in 1940.

Codman had hoped to use the Hospital Standardization Committee to help promote the End Result System, and his fellow committee members supported him in that. An early report from the committee did not mince words. "A factory which sells its products takes pains to assure itself that the product is a good one, but a hospital which gives away its product seems to regard the quality of that product as not worthy of investigation," the committee asserted in 1913. "In a way, trustees of hospitals who do not investigate the results to their patients do not audit their accounts." Although a number of hospitals, including Massachusetts General, adopted some features of the End Result System and a few hospitals adopted virtually all of it, the system as a whole fell

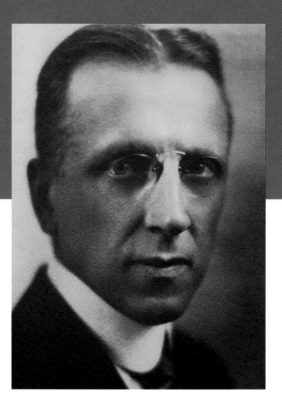

by the wayside. Even if Codman himself had been tactful and politically skilled, however, it is unlikely that the End Result Idea would have gotten much further than it did. The idea was difficult, costly, and threatening to the reputations of both doctors and hospitals. They liked to trumpet success, but preferred to downplay failure. Moreover, practically no incentives existed to implement it. Seventy and eighty years later, when another attempt was made to focus on outcomes research and implementation, incentives were stronger, but it still did not come easily or without struggle.

THE ACS AND THE HOSPITAL STANDARDIZATION PROGRAM

Although Codman's visionary idea sank into obscurity, the idea of hospital standardization was kept alive — and even thrived — thanks to the interest and involvement of the ACS. The case reports of candidates for fellowship in the college in its first years provided a sad commentary on the condition of many hospitals. "Sixty percent of otherwise approved candidates were rejected during the first three years because of poor [hospital] records," Carl P. Schlicke of the ACS wrote. Poor record keeping was just one of several common shortcomings in hospitals.

In 1914, the ACS hired as its first director John G. Bowman, who held a Ph.D. and was the former president of the University of Iowa. The following year — the same year Codman resigned as chairman of the Hospital Standardization Committee — Bowman approached the AMA about taking over the nascent project on hospital standardization, but was turned down because the AMA considered the task too big and too costly. The American Hospital Association (AHA), which had been founded as the Association of Hospital Superintendents in 1899 and changed its name in 1908, offered cooperation, but no money. Codman himself had initially but unsuccessfully tried to interest the Carnegie Foundation in his committee's work. Now Bowman, who previously had been the secretary of the Carnegie Foundation and had good relations with its president, was able to secure a $30,000 grant from Carnegie that underwrote the beginnings of an actual hospital standardization program.

Three hundred ACS fellows along with sixty leading hospital superintendents met in Chicago for a three-day conference in the fall of 1917 to discuss conditions in hospitals and the kinds of improvements that would be necessary to ensure proper care and treatment of patients. This conference established the principle that knowledgeable professionals should assess hospital conditions and endeavor to achieve consensus among themselves on standards that would have the greatest effect on improving patient care. This principle would become fundamental to hospital standardization and later to hospital accreditation.

Following the conclusion of the conference, the ACS board of regents named a 21-member committee to formulate a hospital evaluation questionnaire and to develop a minimum standard. The questionnaire was mailed out to more than 2,700 hospitals in the United States and Canada. The committee decided to postpone publication of its minimum standard, however, until it could be field-tested. The committee expected that at least 1,000 hospitals would meet the standard. Beginning in April 1918, Bowman and his aides conducted field trials. They were hampered first by wartime exigencies and then by the devastating influenza epidemic. The entire standardization effort did get a significant boost in 1919, however, when it won support and a pledge of cooperation from the Catholic Hospital Association of the United States and Canada. An estimated half of all hospital beds in the two countries were in Catholic institutions. Many Catholic hospitals were small community institutions

The Minimum Standard

1. That physicians and surgeons privileged to practice in the hospital be organized as a definite group or staff. Such organization has nothing to do with the question as to whether the hospital is "open" or "closed," nor need it affect the various existing types of staff organization. The word "staff" is here defined as the group of doctors who practice in the hospital inclusive of all groups such as the "regular staff," "the visiting staff," and the "associated staff."

2. That membership upon the staff be restricted to physicians and surgeons who are (a) full graduates of medicine in good standing and legally licensed to practice in their respective states or provinces, (b) competent in their respective fields, and (c) worthy in character and in matters of professional ethics; that in this latter connection the practice of the division of fees, under any guise whatever, be prohibited.

3. That the staff initiate and, with the approval of the governing board of the hospital, adopt rules, regulations, and policies governing the professional work of the hospital; that these rules, regulations, and policies specifically provide:

   (a) That staff meetings be held at least once each month. (In large hospitals the departments may choose to meet separately.)

   (b) That the staff review and analyze at regular intervals their clinical experience in the various departments of the hospital, such as medicine, surgery, obstetrics, and the other specialties; the clinical records of patients, free and pay, to be the basis for such review and analyses.

4. That accurate and complete records be written for all patients and filed in an accessible manner in the hospital—a complete case record being one which includes identification data; complaint; personal and family history; history of present illness; physical examination; special examinations, such as consultations, clinical laboratory, X-ray and other examinations; provisional or working diagnosis; medical or surgical treatment; gross and microscopical pathological findings; progress notes; final diagnosis; condition on discharge; follow-up and, in case of death, autopsy findings.

5. That diagnostic and therapeutic facilities under competent supervision be available for the study, diagnosis, and treatment of patients, these to include, at least (a) a clinical laboratory providing chemical, bacteriological, serological, and pathological services; (b) an X-ray department providing radiographic and fluoroscopic services.

▲ *Franklin Martin and John Bowman drafted the five-point Minimum Standard, which became the basis for the American College of Surgeons' program in hospital standardization and the foundation for all subsequent standards.*

with marginal conditions. By participating in the ACS program, the Catholic Hospital Association could upgrade its institutions and reduce the risk of external control.

During the first half of 1919, Bowman and his staff and members of state standardization committees conducted 20 hospital conferences in the western half of the United States and Canada to explain what the ACS was attempting to do with its standardization program. "As Bowman traveled about the country and as he directed the efforts of the College program," Loyal Davis observed in his history of the ACS, "his well-intentioned presentations were resented as being dictatorial. He was charged with being a schoolmaster who was pedantic and who did not really attempt to see the viewpoint of others." Outside intervention of any kind often was suspect among hospitals, but Bowman did his best to appeal to the hospitals' enlightened self-interest. By adhering to the standards, he advised, they could build goodwill and attract private patients and community donations.

At a conference that preceded another Clinical Congress of Surgeons in New York City on October 24, 1919, Bowman announced the dramatic and shocking results of the field trials. Of the 692 hospitals of 100 beds or more that had been surveyed to date, only 89 had met all of the minimum standards that the ACS had used as its baseline. Only 264 hospitals held regular staff meetings, and only 301 hospitals had case records of patients they treated. A list of the 89 approved hospitals had been printed by the staff with the expectation that it would be distributed, but on the night before the conference was held, the regents of the ACS decided to suppress the list. They feared that it would fall into the hands of the press and embarrass the many prestigious hospitals that had failed to make it. Although the aggregate numbers were announced at the conference, the list of approved hospitals was burned at midnight in the furnace of the Waldorf-Astoria Hotel, eliminating all record of the hospitals on either side of the standard.

The list's incineration was later called an act of intellectual and moral cowardice, but the numbers alone were enough to shock the medical world and to advance the cause of standardization. Franklin Martin and John Bowman quickly collaborated on drafting and publishing the minimum standard. It had only five points: (1) that physicians and surgeons with hospital privileges be organized as a definite group of staff, though it allowed various types of staff organization; (2) that staff membership be restricted to graduates of medical schools in good standing and who were licensed, competent, and worthy in character and in matters of professional ethics (fee-splitting, in which doctors paid other doctors for referrals out of patient fees, was specifically prohib-

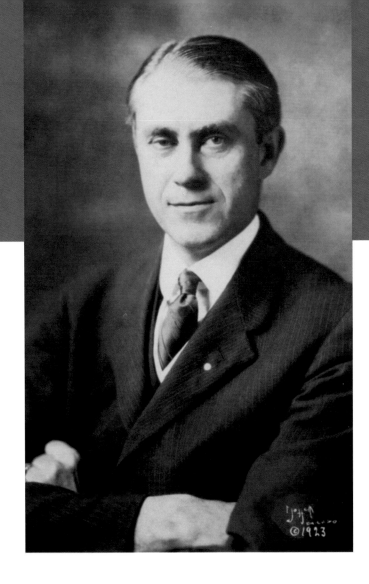

ited); (3) that the staff initiate and, with the approval of the hospital's governing board, adopt rules, regulations, and policies governing the professional work of the hospital, including requirements that staff meetings be held at least monthly and that the staff review and analyze at regular intervals the clinical experience of departments; (4) that accurate and complete case records be written for all patients and filed in an accessible manner in the hospital; and (5) that diagnostic and therapeutic facilities, including a clinical laboratory and an x-ray department, under competent supervision be available for the study, diagnosis, and treatment of patients.

The minimum standard became the basis for the program in hospital standardization, which was soon formally adopted by the regents of the ACS. Impressed with these initial efforts, the Carnegie Foundation made a three-year grant of $25,000 per annum to support the program. The ACS had to come up with the money to match the grant each year. Perhaps tired of criticism from the field, Bowman resigned from the directorship at the end of 1920 and returned to academia, becoming chancellor of the University of Pittsburgh. A Utah judge succeeded Bowman but resigned after a few months. Nevertheless, the ball was rolling.

In May 1920, *Surgery, Gynecology & Obstetrics* reported that the hospital standardization program had seven doctors in the field doing hospital evalua-

tions and that they had been instructed "to collect facts...not [be] a detective...to be helpful and constructive." As the earlier reactions to Bowman had indicated, from the program's beginning, a tension existed between inspection (snooping, approving, or disapproving) and education (helping, advising, teaching). The following January, the ACS reversed course and began to publish a list of hospitals that had met the minimum standard. In 1920, 29 percent of 100-bed hospitals met the standard. In 1921, the approval rate rose dramatically to 76 percent and in 1922 to 83 percent. The ACS also began to survey medium-size hospitals, those with 50 to 99 beds, and in 1922 it

AMERICAN COLLEGE OF SURGEONS

MANUAL OF HOSPITAL STANDARDIZATION

HISTORY, DEVELOPMENT, AND PROGRESS OF HOSPITAL STANDARDIZATION

THE American College of Surgeons, founded in 1913 by surgeons of the United States and Canada, is the originator of Hospital Standardization. The desire of the College to advance the practice of surgery was directly responsible for the beginning of this movement. In order that surgery might be placed on a higher, more ethical plane, the College established as one of the major requirements for admission to fellowship that each candidate submit one hundred medical records of patients upon whom he had operated, as evidence of surgical judgment and technical ability. Few candidates, however, could comply with this requirement inasmuch as hospitals in the United States and Canada seldom kept records which provided accurate data. It was also discovered that the average hospital lacked laboratory, x-ray, and other essential diagnostic and therapeutic facilities necessary to the surgeon in making a proper preoperative study of his patient. Furthermore, medical staffs of hospitals were not organized and the professional work generally lacked supervision; most hospitals were deficient from the standpoint of scientific efficiency. The need for improvement was evident.

After several years of preliminary study and investigation, which included surveys of many hospitals and consultations with eminent authorities and officers of national organizations, the epoch-making program in hospital and medical history, known as Hospital Standardization, was inaugurated in 1918. This program, sponsored and financed by the American College of Surgeons, was received with interest beyond all expectation by the hospitals of the United States and Canada. The growth of the movement has been constant and substantial and now its influence extends to foreign countries, where many institutions are applying the principles advocated, which insure efficient and scientific care of the patient. There are now, at the close of the twenty-eighth annual survey, more than 60,000 reports on file which show definite and encouraging evidence of progress by hospitals in the fulfillment of their obligations to their ill and injured patients.

HOSPITAL STANDARDIZATION DEFINED

Hospital Standardization is a movement to encourage all hospitals to apply certain fundamental principles for the efficient care of the patient which are set forth in the Minimum Standard for Hospitals. Its object is to promote better hospitalization in all its phases in order to give the patient the greatest benefits that medical science has to offer. Throughout the history and development of Hospital Standardization a definite theme has been sounded, namely, *the proper care of the sick and injured*. Its aim is to create in the hospital an environment which will assure the best possible care of the patient. What this means to hospital progress is apparent when one realizes that the standardization program requires that each hospital which qualifies for approval shall have an organized, competent, and ethical medical staff; that the staff shall hold regular conferences for review of the clinical work; that fee-splitting shall be prohibited; that accurate and complete medical records shall be written for all patients treated; and that adequate diagnostic and therapeutic facilities, including a clinical laboratory and x-ray department, shall be provided. This involves facilities, personnel, and procedures predicated upon efficient organization, progressive management, and competent personnel imbued with a scientific and humanitarian spirit. When an institution adopts and successfully applies the above named principles, which express the high standards of modern medical and hospital practice, it is known as a standardized or approved hospital. These fundamental principles, which are readily adaptable to all institutions caring for the sick, are

5

In 1926, the American College of Surgeons published its first Manual of Hospital Standardization. *It was 18 pages long.* The American College of Surgeons made the three-story former residence shown opposite, on Chicago's rapidly growing north side, its headquarters in 1920.

reported that only 43 percent of those had met the minimum standard.

In view of the results, Franklin Martin, who had become director of the ACS, exulted in 1924 that "this document has now achieved international fame, and has become to hospital betterment what the Sermon on the Mount is to a great religion." The year before, in 1923, Malcolm T. MacEachern became associate director of the ACS and took over administration of the

hospital program. MacEachern was a Canadian obstetrician who had been superintendent of Vancouver General Hospital for nine years and then had spent a year traveling across the country surveying nursing conditions. After he moved to ACS headquarters in Chicago, he solidified the program and directed it for the next 28 years. He was an enthusiastic ambassador for it throughout the United States and Canada. He became a powerful figure in hospital administration and also served on many committees of the American Hospital Association. Following his retirement from the ACS in 1951, he wrote the basic text in hospital administration and directed Northwestern University's program in hospital administration.

The hospital standardization program enhanced the stature and credibility of the ACS itself. "The ACS presented itself in the 1920s as a private organization engaged in establishing voluntary standards for hospitals in the interests of patients," historian Rosemary Stevens observed. "Certification under the standardization plan was conveniently analogous to a 'Good Housekeeping Seal of Approval,' another voluntary program for producers and consumers that was developed in the 1920s." Hospitals proudly displayed certificates of approval in their lobbies and sent press releases about receiving them to local newspapers. ACS meetings, rather than those of the AHA or the AMA, provided forums in the 1920s for discussion and debate about critical questions of

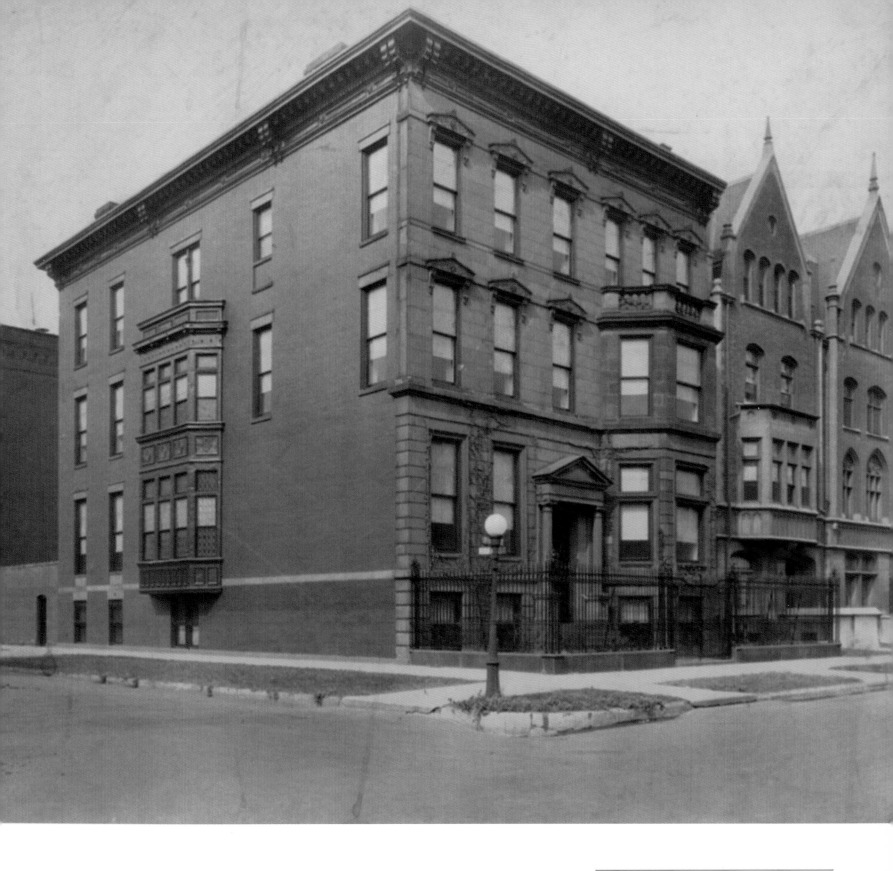

hospital management. Scientifically, the standardization program helped focus surgery on pathological findings, while elevating the importance of laboratories and accuracy in diagnosis in all hospitals.

The standardization program began but it certainly did not end with the minimum standard. Notably, in 1926, the ACS published its first *Manual of Hospital Standardization*. Its 18 pages explained and extended each principle. The manual also contained a statement on the "By-Products of Standardization," which was based on 13,360 surveys that had been conducted over the preceding nine years. It highlighted such things as better organization, facilities, personnel, and coordination and also claimed but did not document improved end results in patient care. The manuals, which were printed and distributed by the thousands, became the bible for every hospital administrator seeking ACS approval. The manuals were revised every several years and grew through additional explanatory sections. The 1946 edition had 118 pages, an increase of 100 pages in 20 years. In 1949, a point rating system was initiated. A perfect score was 900 points, made up of 640 "essential points" and 260 "complementary points."

The ACS employed a staff of inspectors, all of whom were physicians and many of whom were ACS fellows. Most were full-time employees, and they led a peripatetic life, moving from town to town as their work required. Periodically they gathered at ACS headquarters in Chicago for briefings and critiques. In the 1920s, the ACS deliberately chose as inspectors fairly recent medical graduates, who were better-trained and more attuned to recent medical advances. Their relative youth and inexperience sometimes raised the hackles of older practitioners in the field.

Although the Carnegie Foundation had provided seed capital for the program when it began, the financial burden soon fell entirely on the ACS. In 1941, the program's operating budget was $44,000; eight years later it had grown to $68,500. The entire budget came from dues paid to the ACS by its members. In 1950, a total of 3,290 hospitals were on the approved list, representing half the hospitals in the United States. The hospital standardization program was the ACS's largest annual expenditure and made it difficult for the ACS to develop other programs in which it was interested. Demand for the hospital standardization program was only going to grow. In 1946, Congress had passed the Hill-Burton Act, providing federal funding for hospital construction throughout the country. The complicated funding formula favored applications from rural areas and poorer states, many of which were in the South. Although Hill-Burton funding was slow to be appropriated at first, over its first 20 years, 4,678 construction projects received federal funding, almost half in communities with populations under 10,000. Hill-Burton stipulated that hospitals receiving funding have ACS certifica-

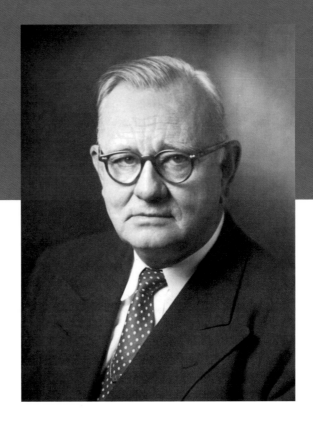

tion. Through this stipulation, the government validated the private sector contribution of the ACS to hospital standardization and certification.

FINANCIAL STRAINS AND THE SEARCH FOR A NEW SPONSOR

In 1950, the regents of the ACS named Paul R. Hawley director, its first since the death of Franklin Martin 15 years before. In the intervening years, the ACS had operated with two associate directors, one of whom was MacEachern. Because of financial difficulties, the ACS eliminated the other associate director position in 1949 and made MacEachern director, but only until a permanent replacement could be found. Arthur W. Allen, the highly capable Boston-based chairman of the ACS board of regents, believed that Hawley was the right man. After graduating from medical school, Hawley had practiced briefly with his father, a country doctor in Indiana. He had joined the U.S. Army Medical Corps during World War I and had spent most of his career in the army, rising in rank to major general. During World War II, he served as the surgical head of the European theater of operations. After the war, when General Omar Bradley became head of the Veterans Administration, Bradley named Hawley its chief medical director. When Bradley left the VA, Hawley also resigned. He became chief executive officer of the Blue Cross-Blue Shield Commission before being named director of the ACS.

Shortly after Hawley took over as director, he learned that the college would be in the red that year unless it shed some major expense. The hospital standardization program was the obvious candidate for shedding, and MacEachern suggested that the logical organization to take it over was the American Hospital Association. Hawley himself had had favorable relations with the AHA when he was at the VA. In fact, ACS relations with the AHA had historically been better than its relations with the AMA, the other likely candidate. With the permission of the regents, Hawley approached George Bugbee, the AHA's executive director. Bugbee was enthusiastic about the idea, and he soon reported that the AHA board liked it as well. Under Bugbee, the AHA had become a much stronger organization and a significant lobbyist for hospital interests in Washington. In the past, the AHA had been frustrated that the ACS standardization program did not pay enough

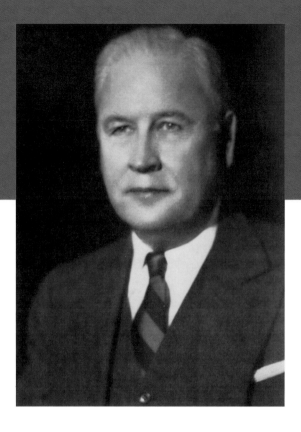

attention to the non-medical aspects of running hospitals and had therefore considered establishing its own program. In preliminary conversations with Hawley, AHA trustees told him that they were prepared to provide an annual budget of $100,000 for a hospital program.

By the summer of 1950, a draft agreement had been drawn up for the program's transfer to the AHA. But the AMA, which had gotten wind of this agreement, disliked the idea of the program being turned over to "laymen" or "civilians," as doctors generally viewed hospital administrators and trustees. The AMA had an accreditation program for internships and residencies and depended on the ACS to certify hospitals. Fearing a loss of clinical control, the AMA dreaded an AHA takeover. In August, a high-ranking delegation from the AMA met with Arthur Allen, three ACS regents, and Paul Hawley to protest the imminent transfer of the pro-

gram to the AHA. The AMA representatives offered to support the program financially or to take it over themselves. They wanted to unite with the ACS against hospital administrators and trustees, who could not be trusted in their view. They were initially unenthusiastic about a suggestion for a cooperative plan that would include the AMA, the AHA, the ACS, and the American College of Physicians (ACP), which had been founded in 1915. A specialist society for internal medicine, the ACP had in recent years taken a particular interest in the training of internists in the hospital environment.

Later that day, the ACS board of regents voted to table the draft agreement with the AHA but to pursue establishment of a cooperative plan that would include the AMA. On the very next day, the AHA trustees expressed disappointment and adopted a resolution to establish a hospital standardization program of its own, in which it hoped other professional organizations would cooperate. But the AMA slowly began to soften up to the idea of a cooperative arrangement, naming a committee to meet with representatives of other organizations.

At the end of September, representatives of the four organizations met for the first time in Washington. "At the first meeting," Maurice J. Norby, an AHA staff member, recalled, "the doctors sat on one side of the table, except the College of Surgeons representatives. They sat on the other side of the table

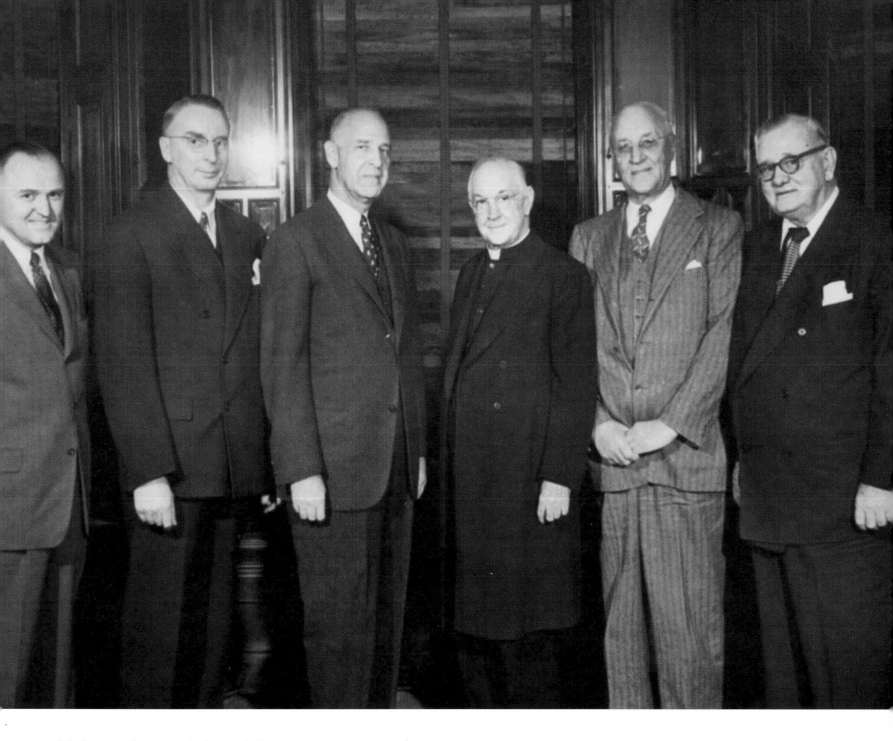

with the American Hospital Association group. Both sides seemed to be glaring at each other. I have never been in such an uncomfortable position."

The negotiations were not easy. "Arthur Allen," writes Loyal Davis, "was always able to point out

In December 1952, Senator Lister Hill, co-sponsor of the Hill-Burton Act, spoke at a formal conveyance ceremony for the Joint Commission on Accreditation of Hospitals. (Left to right, Edwin L. Crosby, Gunnar Gundersen, Lister Hill, Samuel Cardinal Stritch, Evarts A. Graham, Paul R. Hawley.)

enough encouraging progress to obtain agreement for another meeting." The basic argument was over control of the new entity. How many board seats would go to medicine? How many to hospitals? For its part, the AHA was not worried so much about doctors as it was about the AMA and the attitude of the AMA's largest constituency, general practitioners, whom they feared would emasculate or kill the program. Indeed, the AHA welcomed specialist representation through the two colleges. Other issues that had to be resolved included the relationship between the new entity and existing programs of the sponsoring organizations, how standards were to be formulated, how inspections were to be carried out and by whom, and how accreditation was to be determined. Another issue was how to deal with Canadian representation. Three of the organizations, the AHA, the ACS, and the ACP had Canadian members while the AMA did not.

In March, a small negotiating team representing the four organizations hammered out a draft agreement for a joint commission and invited the Canadian Medical Association to participate. Under the agreement, the AHA and the AMA would each have seven seats on the board of commissioners and the two colleges would each have three seats. All the organizations approved the agreement, but at the AMA house of delegates meeting in June, it encountered considerable resistance from the American

Academy of General Practice. It was a strong component of the house of delegates and had sought corporate membership in the Joint Commission itself. The house of delegates empowered the trustees to act, but urged that they seek greater AMA representation and a reduction in AHA representation. At a meeting in July, AHA representatives flatly refused to consider changing the ratio of members, and the AMA relented. (The AMA placated the American Academy of General Practice by naming a general practitioner to one of its board seats.)

JOINT COMMISSION START-UP

An interesting change in nomenclature occurred between the fall of 1950 and the spring of 1951. In November of 1950, the new entity was to be called the Joint Commission on Hospital Standardization. In the spring, it was called the Joint Commission on Accreditation of Hospitals. There is no record as to why the shift from "standardization" to "accreditation" occurred. It could be that "standardization" had acquired too much of a manufacturing connotation while "accreditation" had a more professional ring. "Accreditation" was, for example, widely used in education. For many people, "accreditation" implied peer-review by professionals. Nevertheless, at the time, "accreditation," "standardization," "certification," "inspection," and "approval" were often used interchangeably.

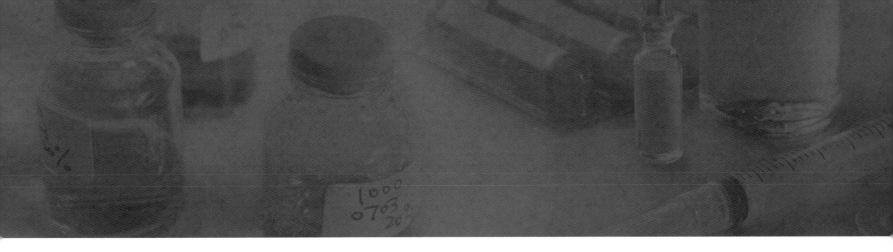

The purpose of the new organization, as summarized by George Stephenson, who wrote a history of the ACS, was "(1) to conduct an inspection and accreditation program that would encourage physicians and hospitals to apply basic principles of organization and administration for efficient care of the patient, promote high quality of medical and hospital care, and maintain diagnostic and therapeutic services through coordinated efforts of staff and governing body in the hospital; (2) to establish standards for hospital operation; (3) to issue certificates of accreditation."

The Joint Commission on Accreditation of Hospitals was incorporated in Illinois in November 1951. It held its first official meeting (an organizational meeting) at the Drake Hotel in Chicago on the morning of December 15, 1951, a Sunday, the preferred meeting day for doctors. All of the corporate members were headquartered in Chicago except for the ACP, which was based in Philadelphia. Gunnar Gundersen, from LaCrosse, Wisconsin, and a member of the AMA, had chaired the earlier meetings and became the commission's first chair that day. Maurice Norby of the AHA made the arrangements. After the breakfast dishes were cleared, waiters walked in with trays containing glasses filled for a toast. Gundersen tried to waive them off, insisting it was a business meeting, but Norby had instructed the waiters to proceed no matter what the chairman said. A California commissioner remarked

that it looked like good California champagne and that as long as it was there, he proposed a toast to the success of the Joint Commission. The commissioners all stood for the toast, tipped their glasses, and sat down with funny looks on their faces. A practical joker, Norby had ordered beer, not champagne.

Norby later recalled that it was "hard for the chairman to get that meeting adjourned. They were complimenting each other, saying great things. Everyone had to make a speech complimenting the other people. They were so happy and pleased. I never have seen such a change in a group. The animosity was completely gone. They were ready to go to work and do a good job." At this meeting, the by-laws were adopted and then immediately amended to include a seat for the Canadian Medical Association. The board elected officers, endorsed the principle that the chairmanship be rotated among the member organizations, discussed arrangements for continuing hospital inspection during the transition, and approved an operating budget of $70,000. The cost was apportioned to member organizations according to the number of board seats, or $3,500 per seat. In like fashion, the organizations agreed to contribute to a reserve fund totaling $25,000.

Malcolm MacEachern's contributions to the hospital standardization program were formally recognized, and the board agreed on the qualifications that it was seeking in the commission's first director. The

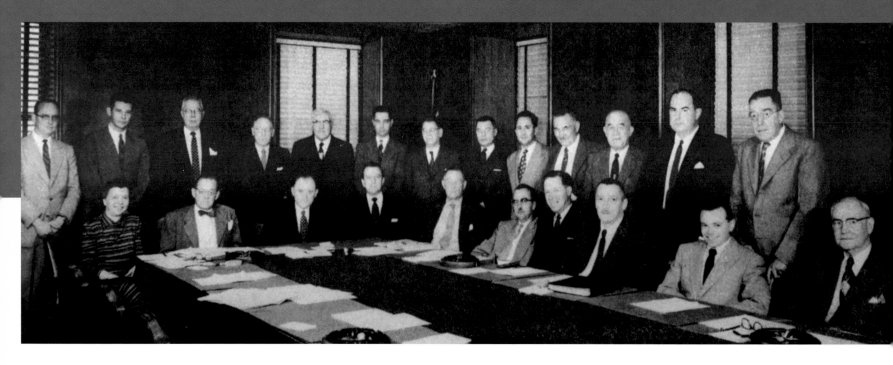

by-laws required that the director be an MD, and the board wanted a physician who was experienced in hospital administration, someone with "demonstrated ability and diplomacy in dealing with both hospital governing boards and physicians on hospital staffs." It turned out that the first choice for the job was present that day, Edwin L. Crosby, president-elect of the AHA. Crosby was very personable, well-liked, and highly respected. He had a medical degree, but he never saw himself as a practicing physician — he liked to say that he would not even treat someone's cat. The Joint Commission has never deviated from the dual medical and administrative qualifications that Crosby had. All of Crosby's successors have been doctors who had then gone into administration. It has been a way for the Joint Commission to try to bridge the historic division between practicing physicians and hospital administrators.

Crosby's parents were in the Salvation Army, and he had gone into public health following medical school. After doing graduate work in public health at Johns Hopkins, he had entered hospital administra-

▲ This photo shows the staff of the Joint Commission on Accreditation of Hospitals in 1954, including "field representatives." Front, left to right: Martha Johnson, Walter E. Batchelder, Edwin L. Crosby, Edward Leveroos, Charles C. Hedges, Joseph R. Anderson, Arthur Springall, Thure A. Nordlander, David L. Robinson, Oliver B. Zeinert. Back left to right: Warren Von Miller, William E. Eaton, Robert S. Meyers, Jose Gonzalez, Fank W. Ryan, William W. Southard, Fernald C. Fitts, William R. Albus.

tion and had risen to be executive director of the highly prestigious Johns Hopkins Hospital. Crosby's career, from public health to hospital administration, tracked the expanding community mission of hospitals themselves. Crosby at first dismissed the idea of becoming director of the Joint Commission, but he changed his mind, perhaps because of the opportunity it offered to influence the entire hospital field. At the next board meeting in March 1952, Crosby was approved as director at a salary of $25,000.

As far as standards and accreditation were concerned, little changed after the Joint Commission

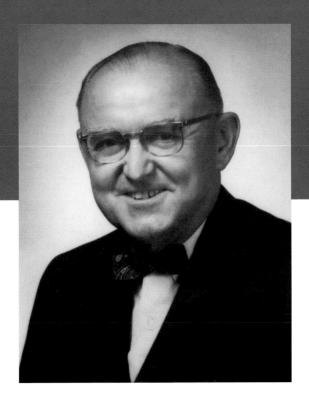

took over from the ACS except that accreditation came from the Joint Commission rather than the ACS. The Joint Commission "grandfathered" all hospitals in 1953 that had already been approved. The point system that the ACS had initiated remained the basis for accrediting new hospitals. The board was determined to act slowly before making any changes in the basic standards. The Joint Commission even remained in the standardization program's former space at ACS headquarters at 660 North Rush Street. The Joint Commission paid rent in the form of a credit on ACS dues. Thus, the only thing that actually changed after the Joint Commission took over was sponsorship.

Crosby assumed the directorship in September 1952 and hired Martha Johnson as his assistant. A registered nurse, with bachelor's and master's degrees in public health, Johnson had most recently been assistant director of the Johns Hopkins School of Nursing. In November, the Joint Commission began publishing its quarterly *Bulletin*, initially a four-page newsletter for communicating with hospitals. Twenty-thousand copies were mailed out to hospital administrators and chiefs of medical staffs in all registered hospitals in the United States and Canada, as well as to all state and local medical associations, hospital associations, and Blue Cross Plans. A 10-day orientation workshop for surveyors was held in Chicago, also in November. Fourteen field representatives from

the ACS, the AMA, and the AHA were briefed prior to going out and surveying hospitals. During the negotiations, a division of surveying responsibilities had been established, building on programs the corporate parents already had that brought them into hospitals. Thus, the ACS would survey hospitals with cancer facilities, the AMA would survey hospitals with intern and residency programs, and the AHA would survey hospitals that had neither of these programs. "Whatever may have been the original purpose of the program," Paul Hawley told the surveyors, "the only important purpose it now serves is that of insuring the best care of patients possible at the present time, and of improving the quality of this care as rapidly as our knowledge and experience will permit....It is the only purpose common to all the member organizations in the Joint Commission on Accreditation of Hospitals."

In December 1952, a formal, well-attended conveyance ceremony was held in the auditorium of the

Number of Hospitals Surveyed by Each Group — 1953	
American College of Surgeons	283
American Hospital Association	564
American Medical Association	400
American Psychiatric Association	54
Joint Commission	5

American College of Surgeons. Senator Lister Hill of Alabama, the co-sponsor of the Hill-Burton Act, was the featured speaker. He credited the ACS for having exercised its great power over hospitals in the interest of the public and for never having usurped this power in its own interest. Edwin Crosby assured readers of the *Bulletin* that "we will continue the accreditation program with this same 'interest of the public' foremost in our minds...in our hearts...and in our actions."

Six times as many hospitals were surveyed in 1953 than in 1952 when the ACS was still running the program by itself. Altogether, 1,306 hospitals were surveyed in the latter year: 1,202 in the United States, 92 in Canada, and 12 in other countries. Of those surveyed, 1,295 received some kind of accreditation decision: 949 were fully accredited 204 were provisionally accredited, 141 were not accredited, and one had action deferred. The larger the hospital, the greater likelihood of accreditation. Hospitals with

300 beds or more were accredited 99 percent of the time, while those with 25 to 49 beds were accredited 75 percent of the time. (Hospitals with fewer than 25 beds were not surveyed.) The surveys were conducted by 20 field representatives of three of the member organizations plus the American Psychiatric Association, which had been surveying psychiatric hospitals on its own and was in discussions with the Joint Commission about collaborative efforts. The table at left indicates the number of hospitals surveyed by each group.

The *Bulletin* discussed what it meant to be a surveyor, the "eyes and ears" of the Joint Commission. It was above all, a life on the road. One fairly typical surveyor (who obviously was from the ACS) "traveled 25,225 miles by train, plane, and bus. He visited 15 states and Canadian provinces. He surveyed 47 hospitals with cancer facilities and 36 cancer clinics and diagnostic centers. He participated in 95 special conferences. He was away from his home base 244 of the 365 days of 1953." In one six-week period, this particular surveyor concentrated on Florida, Alabama, and Mississippi, where he surveyed 5 hospitals and 25 cancer facilities and attended 30 conferences. Surveyors reported to the Joint Commission on their findings, but it was the board of commissioners that made all decisions on accreditation.

It had been something of a surprise when Crosby took the directorship, so perhaps it was not too sur-

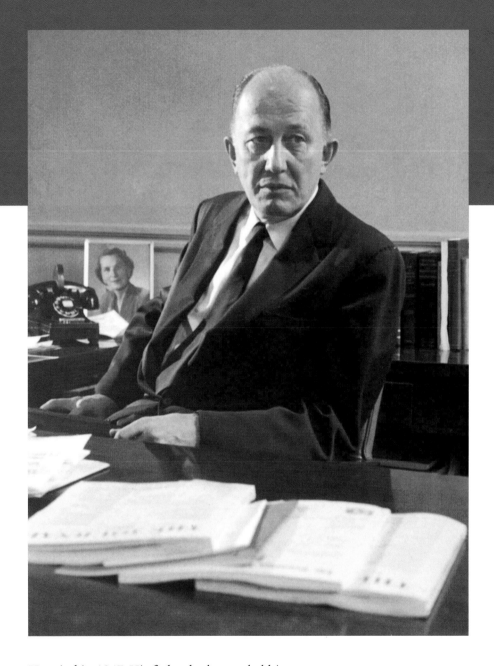

prising that he did not stay long. The Joint Commission in 1953 was, after all, a very small operation. In October 1953, former president Herbert Hoover asked Crosby to serve as research director on a task force on medical services in the federal government. This was part of a commission on organization of the executive branch that Hoover chaired. The board of commissioners agreed to loan Crosby to the government for what was to be part-time work. Then in the spring of 1954, Crosby resigned from the Joint Commission to become executive director (chief executive) of the American Hospital Association, a position he held until his death in 1972. (Martha Johnson stayed on as assistant director at the Joint Commission for a number of years.)

Kenneth B. Babcock succeeded Crosby as director in July 1954. "Dr. Babcock's career, first as a physician and surgeon and then as a hospital administrator, guarantees the sound continuance of this program which got off to such an excellent start," announced Newel W. Philpott of Montreal, the Commission's chairman at that time. Babcock had been an Olympic swimmer in his youth and was a big, energetic, and decisive man. With the exception of military service during World War II, he had spent most of his career at the 900-bed Grace Hospital in Detroit, Michigan. He became a fellow of the American College of Surgeons in 1938, entered hospital administration three years later, and became director of Grace

Hospital in 1947. His father had preceded him as director; together they ran Grace Hospital for a combined 44 years. In 1954, the Joint Commission was on firm ground and in capable hands.

Growth and New Roles

From the perspective of participants today, the Joint Commission in the period from 1955 to 1973 may seem like ancient history and not very relevant. While there are still a few veterans who have memories of the Joint Commission in the early 1970s or before, usually because they were on a hospital staff during surveys, most of those currently involved in the Joint Commission do not go back that far. Recent interviews therefore reveal little about those years. But an interesting story can be extracted from Joint Commission minutes and published sources. It reveals significant developments that have had long-term ramifications.

MODEST CHANGE IN CORPORATE GOVERNANCE

In the mid-1950s, there was an inexorable movement in Canada toward the creation of a separate accreditation organization. The Joint Commission initially bristled at the notion, for three of its corporate members included Canadians within their organizations.

As an organization that was based on voluntarism, however, the Joint Commission obviously could not compel the Canadian Medical Association to stay when it resigned from the Joint Commission, effective December 31, 1958.

By a bare majority, the Joint Commission voted to discontinue surveying Canadian hospitals as soon as the new Canadian Council on Hospital Accreditation was able to assume its responsibilities and to supply its Canadian counterpart with present and past records on Canadian hospitals, Joint Commission standards, survey report forms and other supporting documents. So the separation was amicable and the transition smooth. The two organizations developed a friendly, cooperative relationship, which has continued to the present.

Following the CMA's resignation, the Joint Commission's by-laws were revised. The CMA seat reverted to the AMA, which now had seven seats, on a par with the AHA. Representation on the Joint

Commission was a goal for other organizations as well. In 1957, for example, Kenneth Babcock reported to the board that the American College of Obstetrics and Gynecology and the American Dental Association were seeking membership. In addition, Babcock said that there had been inquiries from the American Academy of General Practice and from organizations of radiologists and pathologists as well. Over the next 16 years, these and other professional groups periodically knocked at the Joint Commission's door.

The Joint Commission's by-laws stipulated that new members could be added with the unanimous consent of the member organizations, but such consent was not forthcoming. The Joint Commission's exclusivity hardly made it popular with the organizations that were denied membership. Over time, however, the Joint Commission included representatives from other professional organizations through a multiplicity of committees, task forces, and categorical councils.

AMA ANXIETIES

The departure of the CMA was not the only thing stirring up the pot. Although the Joint Commission began with a great outpouring of fellowship, it did not take long before AMA doubts and anxieties began to surface. Doctors worried about the possibility that the Joint Commission would become a tough policing body. They feared that accreditation would allow hospital administrators to take control of clinical matters. In 1954, the AMA house of delegates voted to halt any "attempts by hospital accreditation authorities to propose, recommend and by threat of reprisal force the adoption of rules, regulations and various and diverse requirements which would look to the most minute and detailed overlordship in every phase of our hospital practices." This was followed the next year by the creation of a special five-member AMA committee, chaired by Wendell C. Stover, to review Joint Commission functions.

The Stover Committee in June 1956 reported to the AMA house of delegates, which endorsed its report. Although the committee supported accreditation generally and the Joint Commission specifically, it took exception to a number of standards and practices. For example, the Stover Committee said that administrative bodies of hospitals should include physician members. It accepted the Joint Commission requirement that medical staff meetings be held, but objected to the high attendance levels required. The Stover Committee proposed that reports on surveys be sent to both administrators and chiefs of medical staffs, and it proposed that the Joint Commission directly employ and supervise surveyors and that they receive better training.

In the August *Bulletin,* Babcock gave a point-by-point response to each of the report's conclusions, while striking a reassuring tone. On some conclusions,

BULLETIN OF THE JOINT COMMISSION ON ACCREDITATION OF HOSPITALS
660 North Rush Street, Chicago 11, Illinois, Mich. 2-3369

Member Organizations
American College of Physicians
American College of Surgeons
American Hospital Association
American Medical Association
Canadian Medical Association

Edwin L. Crosby, M.D., Director

HISTORICAL
Publications File

November 1952   Vol. 1 - No. 1

Ever since our new office was opened on September 1st---

--- We have been planning the preparation of this initial bulletin, the first in a series that we're going to send to you to keep you informed of the progress of the Joint Commission on Accreditation of Hospitals.

First of all, the address of the Joint Commission is 660 North Rush Street, virtually in the heart of Chicago's Near North Side. The postal zone number here is 11. It's a fine location, quite close to such member associations as the American College of Surgeons, the American Medical Association and the American Hospital Association.

You should know, too, that an assistant to help with the many activities of the Joint Commission has been appointed. She is Martha Johnson, R.N., who has the title: Assistant to the Director. She, also, is located at this office on Rush street.

As you know, the purpose of the Joint Commission on Accreditation of Hospitals is to carry on the hospital standardization program conducted by the American College of Surgeons since 1919. Directing a project that, for so many years, has been superbly handled by this organization is not the easiest assignment.

But the Joint Commission intends to do its best to carry out the program of the ACS. And in this bulletin, you'll find helpful information about the way in which we hope to do it...

One of the first actions taken by the Board of Commissioners of the Joint Commission was the adoption of the program of the American College of Surgeons. In addition, a "Grandfather's Clause" consisting of two parts was established.

The first part of the clause states that the Joint Commission will accredit all hospitals for the year 1953 which, at present, have full approval of the American College of Surgeons.

▲ *The Joint Commission published the first issue of the* Bulletin *in November 1952. The quarterly newsletter was sent to hospital administrators and chiefs of staff nationwide in an effort to improve communication to hospitals.*

such as the principle that the Joint Commission "is not and should not be punitive" and that the present organizational representation on the Joint Commission be maintained, he naturally reported complete agreement. On several other conclusions, Babcock indicated that the Stover Committee's recommendation had been adopted or was being referred to committee for prompt action, including more relaxed medical staff attendance requirements. As for the Stover Committee's insistence that hospital boards be required to include doctors, Babcock explained that the Joint Commission had always encouraged close liaison between hospital governing boards and their medical staffs. However, "the Commissioners think that the composition of the governing board of a hospital should be determined at the local level and that the Commission should not specifically state whether physicians should or should not be members."

Two years later, in 1958, the Joint Commission gingerly entered the troubled waters of medical staff appointments, another contentious issue between medical staffs and hospital governing bodies. Adopting language that had been worked out jointly by the AMA and the AHA, it encouraged hospitals to establish "Joint Conference Committees" as a way of keeping lines of communication open between governing boards and medical staffs. "The governing body," Babcock reported in the *Bulletin*, "has the legal

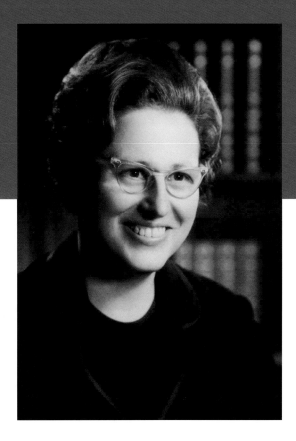

right to appoint the medical staff and the moral obligation to appoint only those physicians who are judged by their fellows to be worthy, of good character, qualified and competent in their respective fields." He noted that one of the most important and difficult responsibilities of a medical staff was selection of doctors and delineation of privileges of individual staff members. "Under no circumstances should the accordance of staff membership or professional privileges be dependent solely upon certification, fellowship or membership in a specialty body or society."

As this statement implies, general practitioners remained wary of elitist specialization. The Joint Commission urged that a hospital medical staff set up a system to select its members and delineate privileges, but it demurred from prescribing exactly what the system or the criteria should be. Above all, a credentials committee must have integrity, Babcock explained. In considering any individual for staff privileges, Babcock suggested that down-to-earth questions be asked: "Would I let this man operate on me or my family for appendicitis, read my electrocardiograms, use hypnotism on me, etc?" If the answer was no, he advised that the doctor in question should not be allowed to treat anyone else.

Since Babcock's hypothetical doctor was a man, it should be noted that the commission was comprised entirely of men until 1973, when Sister Virginia

Schwager, an AHA representative who was a Catholic nun, became the first woman to serve on the board. (Catholic priests had long served on it.)

Discrimination was widespread in society, including medicine and hospitals, but the Joint Commission was virtually silent about it prior to 1970. In August 1963, with a civil rights revolution erupting on the nation's streets, Babcock raised the issue at a board meeting. Board members representing the AMA reported on its attitude on this matter, though it was not recorded in the minutes. The consensus within the board was that the Joint Commission was not violating any civil rights law. The board did take the precaution of deleting a reference in its survey report forms to staff requirements including membership in or eligibility for the local medical society, thereby distancing itself from certain fairly common discriminatory practices.

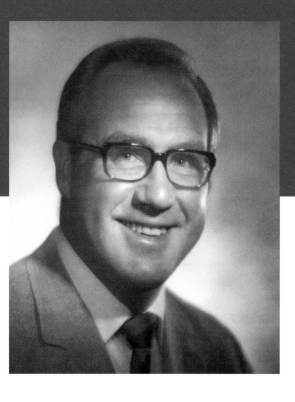

Accreditation standards from 1952 until the late 1960s were essentially those that had been set by the ACS, though they were augmented and amended over the years. As in the days of hospital certification, the principal focus of the survey process was the general fitness of a hospital. The Joint Commission operated on the assumption that if the hospital environment was good, patient care would be good as well and provided a framework for assessing a hospital's administrative structure and resources.

Surveyors looked for evidence of a sound hospital environment, including an organized medical staff, hospital and medical staff by-laws, satisfactory patient records, tissue review, the proper use of autoclaves, mass casualty and disaster plans, as well as professionally staffed x-ray and dietary departments, clinical laboratories and pharmacies. Surveyors evaluated a hospital's physical plant, safety controls, and cleanliness. "The Commission considers fire hazards so serious that no matter how excellent the medical care, a hos-

pital that is a fire trap will not be accredited," Babcock asserted in 1961. Through the *Bulletin* and the survey process itself, the Joint Commission promoted good hospital practices in infection control, blood transfusion services, and drug safety, among other areas.

Babcock as director and the board of commissioners shared responsibility for accreditation decisions and development of standards. After receiving data and observations from surveyors in the field, Babcock, assisted by a small staff, made accreditation decisions, which were usually ratified by the board by mail on a highly pro forma basis. Denver M. Vickers, a reserved doctor who joined the staff in 1955, became assistant director under Babcock. He spent most of his time reviewing and synopsizing survey reports from the field, a task shared by Babcock. When problems arose, one of them would visit a hospital, sometimes to re-survey it.

Babcock was given considerable authority by the board, which convened three times a year in a wood-paneled room of the private Lake Shore Club in Chicago and stayed on for cocktails and dinner afterward. Board meetings were attended by some or all of the executive directors of the member organizations, three of which were based in Chicago. These executive directors, together with Babcock, comprised an Advisory Committee. Ed Crosby, the Joint Commission's first director, served on this committee as the AHA's chief executive officer.

The board of commissioners determined the language of the standards, but Babcock interpreted them for hospitals and surveyors. Like Malcolm MacEachern before him, Babcock became a major figure in hospital administration. He communicated through the *Bulletin*, and he traveled widely and participated in many professional meetings and activities. Elbert Gilbertson, a member of the board of commissioners in the late 1980s, attended Babcock lectures about the Joint Commission when he was a graduate student in hospital administration at the University of Minnesota in the 1950s. Gilbertson recalled Babcock as a "legendary figure" and developed an enormous respect for the Joint Commission as a result of these lectures.

In 1960, the board recommended to its member organizations that they encourage physicians and hospitals to use on a trial basis a method of internal appraisal of medical care, such as one recently proposed by the ACP, or that they institute medical audits. Surveyors looked for evidence that a hospital's medical staff reviewed and evaluated clinical practice, but the commission declined to specify precise methods of medical appraisal or audit. "A review or audit committee must never be rigid or arbitrary," Babcock opined in 1963. "There are honest differences of opinion in the treatment and care of the sick, and these must be honored. The Joint Commission hopes that hospitals will continually, through every possi-

ble means, strive for improved care of patients. The exact mechanisms of how attempts will be made to improve patient care are not as important as the fact that there is intent and desire to do so." The surveys themselves, he liked to point out, were not substitutes for medical audits.

Six years after the AMA adopted the Stover report, unhappiness and suspicion about the Joint Commission surfaced again. In 1962, the Florida delegation to the AMA house of delegates proposed a resolution to bring the Joint Commission within the framework of the AMA — in effect, to scrap its existing organization. Although this particular resolution was tabled, the AMA appointed a new five-member committee to conduct another detailed study of the Joint Commission. The committee, chaired by Thomas W. McCreary, visited the Joint Commission's headquarters, reviewed its operations and procedures, interviewed Babcock, accompanied surveyors to hospitals, and solicited comments, suggestions and criticisms from practicing physicians.

In addition, the committee mailed an opinion survey to administrators and chiefs of staff of 494 hospitals out of the 1,687 hospitals that had been surveyed in 1962. Their responses give a picture of how the Joint Commission was regarded in the field 10 years after its creation. Hospital administrators generally held it in higher regard than physicians did. Half of the administrators but only 28 percent

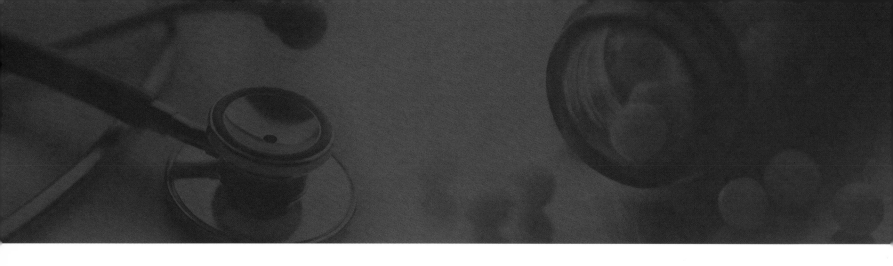

of medical chiefs of staff felt that the Joint Commission's accreditation program had improved patient care a great deal, while 40 percent of administrators and 49 percent of physicians said patient care had improved some, and 10 percent of administrators and 23 percent of physicians felt that it had been responsible for improving patient care very little or not at all. Although 92 percent of administrators and doctors alike indicated that the Joint Commission had assisted their hospitals in maintaining high administrative and professional standards, only 21 percent of physicians and 35 percent of administrators believed that it had improved essential diagnostic and therapeutic services in their hospitals.

In the end, the McCreary Committee, like the Stover Committee, accepted the organizational status quo. The committee found that the Joint Commission emphasized hospital administrative practices and concluded that the commission should review its standards with the goal of emphasizing and strengthening those relating to improved patient care and essential diagnostic and therapeutic services. The Joint Commission endorsed 11 out of 13 recommendations from the McCreary Committee. Although the AMA's anxieties never went away completely, by the early 1960s accreditation had won general acceptance from doctors and wide acceptance and a greater degree of appreciation from hospital administrators.

SHIFT TO FULL-TIME SURVEYORS AND CHARGING FOR SURVEYS

During the Joint Commission's first 10 years, surveys were conducted almost entirely by field representatives of the member organizations, usually in conjunction with hospital visitations for other purposes. ACS representatives would also survey a hospital's cancer clinic, ACP or AMA representatives would look at a hospital's residency or internship program, and AHA representatives would survey for institutional registration. In 1956, the Stover Committee had recommended that the Joint Commission employ and oversee surveyors directly and a subsequent AHA task force reached the same conclusion.

It was a wise suggestion to eliminate difficulties and ambiguities associated with surveyors having to fulfill two different missions. But it was financial considerations that eventually drove the shift to full-time surveyors. The number of surveys increased from 1,202 in 1953 to 1,687 in 1962, leaving the corporate members financially drained. The ACP, which had a smaller budget than the other parent organizations, felt particularly burdened by the rising cost of membership, which amounted to $54,000 — $33,000 for field staff and $21,000 to cover its portion of the Joint Commission's overhead — in 1962. (It is interesting to note that the ACP rejected the American Academy of Pediatrics' offer to assume one-third of the ACP's fees in exchange for one of its seats on the board.)

The introduction of hospital charges guaranteed the Joint Commission's principal revenue source long into the future.

At the end of 1962, 3,947 hospitals in the United States were accredited by the Joint Commission. Accreditation had not only become accepted, but was growing in popularity, so the burden on the corporate members was only going to grow. In fact, the Joint Commission's total budget for 1963 amounted to $389,000, $146,000 for overhead and $243,000 for field staff. In 1962, the Joint Commission's Advisory Committee recommended and the board agreed that the actual costs of surveying would be charged to hospitals, effective January 1, 1964. The board had previously spurned this idea, afraid it might make the surveys less objective or at least appear less objective. But the prospect of relief from the burden of paying the direct costs of surveying ultimately prevailed.

The introduction of hospital charges guaranteed the Joint Commission's principal revenue source long into the future and allowed it to hire, train and manage its own staff of surveyors. These decisions laid the basis for a larger and more robust organization, which could also achieve a greater degree of autonomy from its corporate members over time. The hospitals paid the bills and therefore became the Joint Commission's immediate customers, but the corporate members, only one of which represented hospitals per se, still controlled the Joint Commission, a situation that later would lead to internal tensions.

There was some anxiety about whether hospitals would accept the idea of having to pay for surveys. But hospitals had an economic incentive to go along. They were becoming more dependent on third-party payments from Blue Cross, private health insurers, group health plans, and government. The Kerr-Mills Act of 1960 instituted a program through which states that chose to participate reimbursed hospitals for care of indigent patients. Nearly 68 percent of Americans in 1960 had some hospital insurance, often through Blue Cross. Insurance benefits represented 64 percent of all nongovernmental payments for hospital care in 1960. Most important, third-party payers were not only recognizing Joint Commission accreditation as an indicator of good patient care, but they were beginning to require it as a condition of reimbursement. "The Commission's function is to help hospitals," Babcock explained a bit defensively in 1960. "It is not punitive in character and has no authority to 'make' anyone do anything. The pressures come from other agencies which have recognized that the standards established by the Commission have proved to be effective in assuring safe patient care, and have used accreditation as a criterion for their own purposes."

The new funding system was announced in the December 1962 *Bulletin*. The member organizations would continue to pay administrative overhead, but individual hospitals would be charged for surveys using the following formula: "Beginning January 1, 1964, and thereafter until further notice, the charge for hospital surveys will be $60.00 per hospital, plus

$1.00 per bed (exclusive of bassinets) up to 250 beds. This will mean that the smallest eligible hospital of 25 beds would pay $60.00 plus $25.00, or a total cost of $85.00. A hospital of 250 beds or more would pay $60.00 plus $25.00, or a total cost of $310.00." Hospitals were notified of a survey a month in advance and an invoice was included. They were asked to pay before the survey was conducted. "Whether or not payment has been received, the survey will be made. It is of no concern to the surveyor whether or not payment has been made, and under no circumstances is he to accept the survey charge fee."

At the next board meeting in March, Babcock reported that he had received only one complaint and it was rather mild. A year later, after the charges had gone into effect, he reported that no hospital had cancelled a survey because of the charge. Moreover, the Joint Commission's checking account had grown to the point where money was being transferred to an interest-bearing savings account. In fact, all hospitals paid for surveys in 1964, clear evidence of a market for the service provided by the Joint Commission.

Typically, accredited institutions were general, acute care hospitals, though some specialized in psychiatry or tuberculosis, or provided long-term or rehabilitative care. In 1963, Babcock reported to the board that 62 percent of eligible hospitals were accredited and that 82 percent of all hospital admissions were in accredited hospitals. Between 1954 and 1964, the total number of accredited hospitals had increased from 2,900 to 4,287. This increase was all the more impressive in view of Canada's withdrawal from the program during these years.

In fact, demand for surveys was straining the Joint Commission's capacity. "Many hospitals apply for an accreditation survey and then do not understand why they have to wait from six months to a year before a survey can be made," Babcock reported in the *Bulletin* in 1963. He explained that the Joint Commission had only 16 surveyors to cover 50 states, plus Puerto Rico and military hospitals abroad. In the 1950s, the Joint Commission had occasionally been asked to accredit foreign hospitals, including some in the Middle East, where Babcock conducted surveys. Aloysio de Salles Fonsecca, a prominent Brazilian physician, has recalled a visit by a team of surveyors from the Joint Commission in 1955 to the Hospital sos Servidores do Estado (HSE) in Rio de Janeiro, which was considered the best hospital in South America. This team reaffirmed the Class A certification that a team from the American College of Surgeons had awarded HSE in 1949.

By 1962, the Joint Commission had accredited hospitals in six countries other than the United States, but it had also decided not to accredit any more foreign hospitals because of a shortage of personnel. Each surveyor had to conduct from 110 to 130 surveys annually, depending on the size of the hospital and the amount of travel required. Hospitals of 200 beds or fewer took one day to survey; 200 to 400 beds took two days, and more than 400 beds required three days. Except for travel outside the contiguous 48 states, surveyors used their own automobiles, with Southern states being surveyed in the winter and Northern states in the summer, to reduce the risk of travel problems. A surveyor's schedule had to be drawn up months in advance.

In 1964, the starting salary of surveyors was $11,000, with a $500 annual increment, up to a maximum salary of $13,000. At the end of the year, the board voted to increase the starting salary to $13,000, with a $500 annual increment, up to a maximum of $15,000. This brought the starting salary into line with what the ACS was currently paying its surveyors of cancer programs. In March 1965, the Joint Commission board authorized a 10 percent transfer of funds from the surveyors' account to the administrative account. Thus, in addition to covering the direct costs of surveying, the fees soon began to contribute to commission overhead. For 1966, this contribution was approximately $34,000, but the figure would grow subsequently.

CHANGE IN LEADERSHIP

Babcock resigned from the directorship in 1964. He was 62, but he did not retire when he resigned. He moved to Florida and worked for a number of years as a consultant to hospitals. It seems possible that Babcock's resignation was welcomed, if it was not actually sought, by the board of commissioners. Jean Gayton Carroll, who joined the staff in a research capacity in 1965, recalls discussion that Babcock had alienated the board by assuming too much personal authority. The Joint Commission had outgrown its space at the ACS, and Babcock sought offices separate from any of the corporate parents. Reportedly, he signed a lease on new office space at 201 East Ohio Street without first consulting the board, though he did get approval from the Advisory Committee. The Joint Commission moved to these offices at the end of 1964.

At the March 1964 board meeting, Babcock recommended that his successor have both clinical and administrative experience, that he be young enough to be able to serve 10 years on the job, and that he have "firmness of character and the ability to say 'yes' and 'no' and still be a diplomat." Babcock recommended the appointment of a second assistant director, arguing, "at present the Director is so hampered by the mechanics of the operation and traveling that

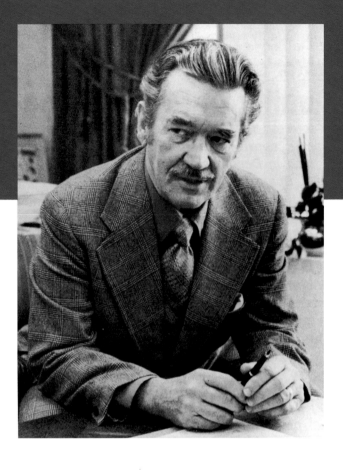

there is no opportunity for creative thinking or even the simplest of research." In addition to making administrative recommendations, he offered some observations, reflections of his accumulated frustrations with the board or its member organizations. "Over the past eleven years," Babcock said, "the Commissioners have eased or lowered Standards in many respects. This is not a criticism — just an observation. The Commissioners have lowered the meeting requirements, requirements of physician assistants at operation, requirement of serology tests, chest x-rays, indexes in pathology and radiology."

In an apparent allusion to frequent AMA criticism, Babcock noted, "accreditation should not be considered a device which will insure control of the medical staff, but rather a means to insure that the medical staff are controlling the activities in the hos-

pital which are concerned with medical and patient care." The job of managing the Joint Commission has never been easy. Arrows fly in from many directions and often hit the Joint Commission's director, who over time accumulates scar tissue. In his pointed farewell observations, Babcock fired a few back.

As it turned out, it took more than a year to find a new director and get him in place. Babcock's resignation became effective in October 1964, at which time Denver Vickers became acting director. The search committee originally selected a senior military officer, who withdrew from consideration five days after his interview (though he later served on the board as an AHA representative). Finally, on June 15, 1965, John D. Porterfield III, who had been chosen in March, took over the reins.

A native of Chicago, Porterfield had graduated from the University of Notre Dame and had received his medical degree from Rush Medical College. Porterfield had not been a clinician but prior to joining the Joint Commission had a distinguished career in public health administration. He had been director of the Ohio State Department of Health from 1947 to 1954 and director of the Ohio Department of Mental Health and Correction for two years before his selection as deputy surgeon general of the U. S. Public Health Service. Prior to joining the Joint Commission, he held an academic appointment at the University of California, Berkeley. Porterfield was president of the American Public Health

Association during 1963 and 1964. He had lectured at many universities and published widely.

Jean Gayton Carroll recalled being told by a board member that an important factor in Porterfield's hiring was that he agreed to keep the board informed at all times and to make no major changes without consulting them. When Porterfield was hired, he was offered an annual salary of $37,500, according to the minutes, "with provisions for doing at least a portion of his work at his home in California, with his intent to move to Chicago as soon as possible." Porterfield rented a small apartment in Chicago. He was in Chicago regularly, but he maintained his primary residence in California. For most of his tenure, Porterfield's wife ran a thriving real estate business in San Diego. He spent as much time as he could with her and with his daughter and grandchildren, who were also in California.

Like Babcock, Porterfield traveled extensively to speaking engagements and participated in various professional meetings, conferences, and activities. He wrote articles for professional journals, did trouble-shooting, and occasionally conducted or observed surveys. His job soon came to include representing the Joint Commission in Washington, D.C. With the board's consent, he participated in professional committees, including the chairmanship of the committee that accredited graduate schools of public health. He also consulted with the Agency for International Development on a hospital-construction program in Vietnam. AID reimbursed the Joint Commission for Porterfield's time.

Porterfield was complex and intelligent, and he was a fine writer, editor, and speaker. As might be expected of someone with a background in public health bureaucracies, he was politically adroit and was comfortable with slow, deliberative processes. He kept the board apprised of his many activities, and he avoided getting too far ahead of it. Committees of the board became both more numerous and more involved in the commission's activities during his tenure. Porterfield never defied the board, though Carroll did recall one instance in which he mildly remonstrated a commissioner. During a heated discussion pitting one of the two largest corporate parents against the other, one board member blurted out, "Hell, I am here to represent the AHA [or it could have been the AMA]." "I thought you were here to represent the Joint Commission," Porterfield said quietly.

EXPANSION BEYOND HOSPITALS

Porterfield's hiring coincided with a consensus by the board of commissioners to expand accreditation into inpatient care institutions other than hospitals. Indeed, it seems likely that his background in public health administration was a major factor in his selection.

The idea of expanding beyond its traditional hospital base had been under discussion since the early 1960s. After Russell A. Nelson of the AHA became board chairman, he observed in 1961 that the Joint Commission had succeeded in winning acceptance and had accredited about "70 percent of the eligible acute general hospitals in this country." "What about the future?" he wondered. Should the Joint Commission just fine-tune its existing program, "or should it reach out in expansion to cover research and education in standards of hospital care and/or enter other fields for accreditation?"

A modest research effort on the quality of care was soon authorized under the chairmanship of Jack Masur, an AHA commissioner who was also an administrator with the National Institutes of Health. This effort was undertaken in collaboration with the University of Pittsburgh. Research had not been a central part of the Joint Commission's mission, and this early research endeavor did not gain much traction. But program expansion did emerge as a priority in the early and mid-1960s. The Joint Commission's very success in the hospital field made it seem logical and proper to expand beyond hospitals. Thanks in no small measure to the example set by the Joint Commission, accreditation was a growing phenomenon in the health field. Voluntary accreditation programs had been developing in specialized areas, such as one for clinical laboratories that had been estab-

lished by the College of American Pathologists or one established by the American Association of Medical Clinics for its members. Meanwhile, accreditation programs were proliferating around skilled nursing homes and residential care facilities, though these programs were fragmented and only regional in scope.

"Recognising these trends, but without wishing arbitrarily to preempt the field of voluntary standards and accreditation," John Brewer, a veteran commissioner from the ACS, explained in a 1971 article, "JCAH moved in 1965 to offer its prestige, experience and expertise in order to encourage a more rational and effective approach for the accreditation of health facilities and services." Since doctors and acute care hospitals were at the top of the professional and institutional hierarchies in health care, it is understandable that their representatives were ready to assist those who came behind them in "prestige, experience and expertise." Some viewed Joint Commission expansion as an expression of self-confidence and good citizenship; others viewed it as an expression of the arrogance of doctors and hospitals.

Although the board was interested in expansion, it did not want to grow at the expense of the hospital program or add to administrative overhead, which was still borne primarily by the corporate members. Tricky political issues took several years to resolve. For example, the American Nursing Home

Association was wary of coming under AHA control. In 1963, the ANHA entered discussions with the AMA about creating a new accrediting body for nursing homes apart from the Joint Commission, and a new organization was soon in the offing. Meanwhile, the AHA had also started its own extended care approval program. Within the AMA, in addition to wariness about the AHA, there was sentiment that nursing homes were different from hospitals in important ways, including the procedures carried out, length of stay and the much higher ratio of proprietary ownership to be found there. If the Joint Commission were to proceed, how would differences between skilled nursing facilities and homes for the aged be treated? Would new standards be established for non-hospital settings and who would write them? If the Joint Commission accredited extended care facilities, would the board be expanded?

It may not be coincidental that these questions began to be resolved shortly after Porterfield assumed the directorship. At the first board meeting he attended as director, in August 1965, the board "expressed its intent to initiate a program of accreditation for extended care facilities at the earliest possible date" and charged him with developing the program. At the next board meeting, in October, Porterfield reported that "much had been accomplished with regard to the work of setting standards for extended care facili-

ties." Grants from the Hartford Foundation, which came through the AHA, underwrote the expense of launching the new program, including hiring staff and developing a set of appropriate standards. But at the outset, standards were simply adopted from programs already in the field.

The scope and infrastructure of the Joint Commission expanded a great deal during Porterfield's tenure, and he gave subordinates considerable running room. Harris B. Jones became assistant director of the Joint Commission in 1965 and was the director of the extended care program into the 1970s. Meanwhile, Otto Arndal, a physician and former surveyor, was soon named a deputy assistant director. In 1966, Arndal became director of the hospital accreditation program when Denver Vickers retired. Arndal emphasized the survey visit as a consultative/educational experience and he strove to improve the quality and training of surveyors. With surveyor salaries low in comparison to compensation in private practice, Arndal recruited many retired military doctors as surveyors. In addition, Porterfield hired Bruce B. Sanderson in 1965 as assistant director for central administration. He resigned in 1968, but administrative positions continued to expand together with the Joint Commission's growth.

In a departure from past policy, the Joint Commission board was expanded in 1965 to include two additional representatives with regular three-year

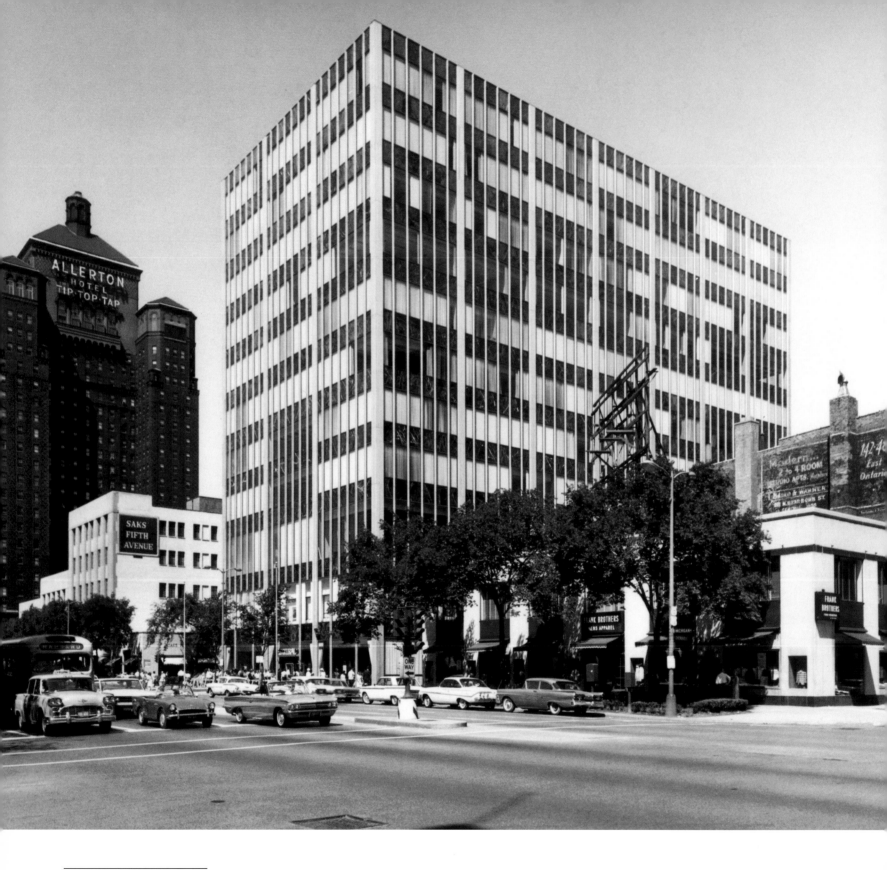

terms, one from the American Association of Homes for the Aging and one from the American Nursing Home Association. Both associations were denied corporate membership but they contributed to overhead at an equivalent rate to other board seats. Since the board had been expanded to 22 seats, each association contributed 1/22 to administrative overhead for each board seat it held. As in the hospital program, fees charged to surveyed institutions financed the extended care program. These fees were lower than hospital fees because the surveys were less expensive. The surveyors, who were all registered nurses, received lower compensation, $9,000 in 1966 compared to $13,000 for physician-surveyors in the hospital program.

The addition of the extended care program, which began operations on January 1, 1966, and the anticipation of further expansion necessitated a move to larger offices in the Blair Building at 645 North Michigan Avenue. This space had been leased by the National Council for the Accreditation of Nursing Homes, the nascent organization that terminated its programs when the Joint Commission entered the field. More than a year after completing this move, the Joint Commission found a tenant to assume the lease at East Ohio Street. Within a few years, the extended care program was being referred to as the long-term care program, which it has remained.

At the end of 1966, the board approved a second major program expansion. In this case, the Joint Commission entered into a contract with the newly formed Commission on Accreditation of Rehabilitation Facilities (CARF), which offered accreditation services to rehabilitation centers, sheltered workshops and organized programs for the homebound. The director of the Joint Commission became the director of CARF. Charles Caniff, the long-time executive director of the Association of Rehabilitation Centers, who had been the interim director of CARF, became assistant director of the Joint Commission and was put in charge of this program. It operated out of the Joint Commission's offices, beginning in early 1967.

This contractual relationship was the model for further growth over the next several years. Through so-called "categorical councils," the board entered into memoranda of agreement with a number of health care organizations other than acute care hospitals. Grants and contracts from the federal government were instrumental both in establishing the need for these new accreditation services and in helping to launch them. Thus, the Joint Commission established the Accreditation Council for Services for the Mentally Retarded and Other Developmentally Disabled Persons in 1969, the Accreditation Council for Psychiatric Facilities in 1970 and the Accreditation Council for Long Term

Care in 1971. The latter council replaced the program that had been established within the regular Joint Commission framework. When it was established, the two representatives who had been added to the board from nursing home associations went off the Joint Commission board and onto the new council.

Each council was required to have sufficient funds in hand to support the first two years of operation. Subsequently, each council's field survey program was expected to generate sufficient income to support operations. Contributions from council members would support each council's overhead. In addition, the memoranda of agreement provided that the councils would contribute 10 percent of their gross survey fee income to support the budget of the Joint Commission's division of research and education.

Although expansion was exciting, it also was difficult. The new programs sometimes struggled to find customers and therefore struggled financially. Turf battles occurred because facilities often offered more than one kind of service. For example, acute care hospitals also frequently offered long-term, psychiatric, or rehabilitation services. Which standards would apply — those of a particular council or those of the hospital accreditation program?

After much debate, the Joint Commission adopted an "all or none principle," which addressed this ques-

tion, but did not completely resolve it. The Joint Commission's corporate members began to feel that the councils were out of control, while the councils grew indignant at what they perceived to be the arrogance of corporate members. Beginning in 1967, the Joint Commission board periodically took up the question of renaming the organization to reflect its broader scope only to table or vote down the idea. The repeated rejection left the non-hospital providers feeling like second-class citizens. In 1971, CARF asked to renegotiate its contract. When these negotiations failed to resolve underlying differences, CARF formally separated from the Joint Commission. CARF moved out of the Joint Commission's offices by the end of that year. So this particular relationship proved short-lived.

ADVENT OF A MORE LITIGIOUS ENVIRONMENT
In 1963, two podiatrists in Washington, D.C., brought suit against Doctors Hospital, a 300-bed proprietary hospital, and against the Joint Commission, charging them with restraint of trade. The hospital had been non-accredited and one of the faults found with it had been that it had two podiatrists on its staff, operating independently and without proper supervision from the medical staff. In its efforts to restore accreditation, the hospital had notified these podiatrists that they could no longer operate independently. The podiatrists, who had

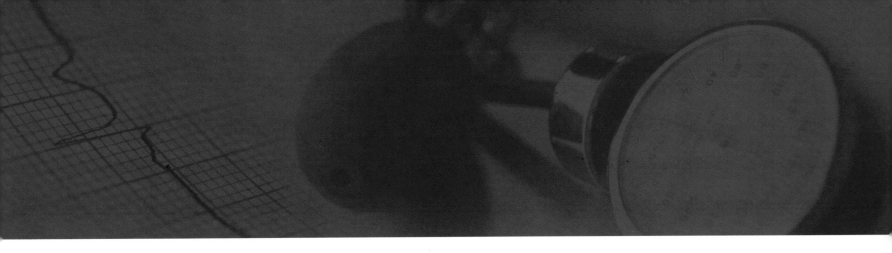

been on the hospital's staff for 20 years, then filed suit. After hearing the Joint Commission's lawyer outline both the favorable and unfavorable aspects of the case, the board authorized him to try to settle it, though without compromising the principle that licensed physicians would oversee patient care in its totality.

The costs of this litigation became worrisome, with legal fees in 1965 exceeding $40,000. This suit and subsequent complaints by podiatrists in California set the Joint Commission on a long process of revising and clarifying standards as they related to podiatrists and other health professionals. Dentists, oral surgeons, osteopaths, psychologists, physical therapists, and nurse midwives, for example, were licensed by individual states to provide care to patients within their disciplines. The litigation by podiatrists was a harbinger of future activism by non-MD health professions to oppose what they viewed as the guild-like restrictions of the medical profession. Through the application of standards in accreditation, the Joint Commission was viewed as an instrument of the medical profession in restricting access to hospitals. The Joint Commission itself became a "dirty name," recalled John Helfrick, who trained as an oral and maxillofacial surgeon in the late 1960s and who 30 years later chaired the Joint Commission.

Another harbinger of a changing environment in 1965 was the *Darling* case, which said that hospitals had a legal responsibility for patient care. In this case, the Supreme Court of Illinois decided in favor of a young football player whose gangrenous leg had to be amputated as a result of deficient treatment in a hospital. Rulings in other state courts, especially in California, were starting to hold hospitals legally and financially responsible for the medical care given by their employees and all affiliated health personnel, including attending physicians. It was becoming much more difficult for hospital administrations to disclaim responsibility for the actions of their professional staff members. Likewise, physicians could no longer so easily claim complete freedom from the hospital's jurisdiction. The old barriers between the civilian and clinical domains in hospitals were much harder to maintain. Not surprisingly, by 1969, the Joint Commission found itself back in the middle of controversy over relationships between governing boards and medical staffs. The AMA house of delegates that year dealt with a barrage of resolutions related to this issue.

MEDICARE WATERSHED

A government program of health insurance had been on the liberal agenda since the 1940s, but the working conservative majority in Congress had long resisted it. Throughout this period of resistance, the AMA had been a powerful lobbyist in Washington and the most prominent voice around the country against any government measure that it construed as "social-ized medicine." But Congressional hearings and print and television reporting periodically exposed glaring shortcomings in the American health care system, especially the precarious situation faced by many older citizens. In 1965, one-half of all Americans older than 65 had no health insurance. Illness and hospitalization could — and not infrequently did — wipe out an elderly person's life savings. By 1965, the AHA and some other health organizations had broken ranks with the AMA and had endorsed the principle of extending social security to include health insurance for the aged.

The landslide election in 1964 of President Lyndon B. Johnson, accompanied by a huge Democratic majority in Congress, broke the logjam on federally financed health insurance for the aged. Johnson, a strong legislative leader, made passage of the Medicare Act his first legislative priority. Public Law 89-97, an amendment to the Social Security Act of 1935, was enacted in June 1965 on a heavily Democratic vote and more than token Republican support.

Under Plan A, Medicare raised social security taxes to subsidize the cost of hospitalization and nursing home care for defined periods of time for people who were at least 65 years of age. Plan B of Medicare was a supplemental insurance program that was supported by government and by payments from recipients of care. It provided reimbursement for certain diagnostic tests, home-nurse visits and doctors' fees. The Medicare legislation also included a Medicaid program, which offered federal matching grants to states that had programs to pay for health care for the poor and indigent.

In the fine print of the Medicare Act was a provision that hospitals accredited by the Joint Commission on Accreditation of Hospitals were "deemed" to be in compliance with most of the *Medicare Conditions of Participation for Hospitals* and thus deemed to meet eligibility requirements for participation in the Medicare program. If a hospital was certified for Medicare, it was also eligible for Medicaid participation. Actually, the ultimate authority to determine whether a hospital met the necessary health and safety requirements was conferred by the Medicare Act upon the secretary of health, education and welfare and the states, except that such requirements could not be higher than those of the Joint Commission. Therefore, the Joint Commission's standards effectively set the ceiling.

How exactly the Joint Commission was included in the Medicare Act remains a mystery. There is no mention of the matter in the Joint Commission's contemporaneous minutes or publications. The Joint Commission had no presence on Capitol Hill at the time, though two of its corporate parents, the AMA and the AHA, did. It seems more likely that the AHA rather than the AMA would have had a hand in the legislative draftsmanship, since the AHA was in better graces with the Johnson administration and with Medicare supporters. The AMA, by contrast, had been Medicare's leading health care opponent.

The inclusion of a role for a private organization in a government-sponsored program had many precedents, including the Hill-Burton program. Moreover, at the time Medicare was enacted, the federal government lacked the administrative capacity to inspect or regulate hospitals. The states lacked this capacity as well, though Medicare stimulated the growth of state licensure agencies. In 1965, the Joint Commission was the only game in town, and it enjoyed wide acceptance and respect. In addition, "deemed status" for the Joint Commission can be seen as part of a larger process of accommodation by the federal government aimed at getting provider participation for the new program. Similarly, officials and lawyers from the U.S. Department of Health, Education and Welfare (HEW) were busy hammering out agreements on reimbursement rules and formulas with Blue Cross and other private representatives. In doing so, they relied heavily on prevailing reimbursement practices in the private sector, which already recognized accreditation by the Joint Commission.

"Deemed status" profoundly affected the Joint Commission. "Suddenly and almost without warning," Carl Schlicke, a board member, reflected in a 1972 speech, "JCAH was catapulted on to the national scene and cast into an entirely new role as a quasi-public licensing body." He added that Porterfield "defined quasi-public as the assumption of all the obligations of public office without the benefits of tax support." Indeed, Medicare opened the Joint Commission to much greater public accountability and criticism. Although those associated with the Joint Commission sometimes muttered about the heavy burden that had been placed on it, no one asked to be relieved of that burden. They all recognized that "deemed status" enhanced the Joint Commission's prestige, influence, and power.

Even though hospitals could get approval for Medicare eligibility through state licensure, a large majority preferred the Joint Commission route. Indicatively, in 1970, 71 percent of U.S. hospitals were accredited by the Joint Commission, while a total of 85 percent were Medicare certified. The Joint Commission was a known quantity, and hospitals and doctors had a strong voice in it through their professional organizations. In 1966, the Joint

One immediate effect of "deemed status" was to stimulate a thorough reexamination of hospital standards.

the field, where standards are, in reality, set, and should be anticipated in the Joint Commission where they may be adopted and promulgated as guidelines for all institutions." In other words, the Joint Commission was essentially in the business of codifying standards that had already been established by leaders in the field.

Porterfield insisted that the Joint Commission's role was educational, not regulatory, and he expected that data gathered from a research program could be utilized effectively in the training of field staff. "Through the use of the products of this program," he said "it is our intention to provide each of our surveyors with the tools necessary to make them the most effective, objective and helpful consultants available to an institution on a one or two day visit." He also hoped that this undertaking would aid in the development of educational programs for administrative and medical personnel in hospitals. Stanley Ferguson, an AHA representative who chaired the Research and Education Committee, reported in December that the first research project was "to cover the review, reevaluation and rewriting of the hospital accreditation standards and their supplemental interpretations, to attain the objectives of raising and strengthening the standards from their present level of 'minimum essential' to the level of 'optimum achievable,' to assure their

Commission tried to get HEW to accord deemed status to its long-term care program, which was struggling because of a lack of business, but was turned down.

REVISION OF HOSPITAL STANDARDS

One immediate effect of "deemed status" was to stimulate a thorough reexamination of hospital standards. "With agencies in every state now certifying hospitals in terms of minimum standards," Porterfield explained to the board in July 1966, "it is possible for the Joint Commission to further the tradition, begun by the American College of Surgeons in 1918 and carried on by the Joint Commission since 1953, of constantly attempting to elevate the quality of care by stepping up to a new plateau. The basis for the identification of this plateau would result from a comprehensive search of our records and perhaps those of other organizations to recognize changing patterns of care. These changing patterns soon become identifiable as moving frontiers of practice in

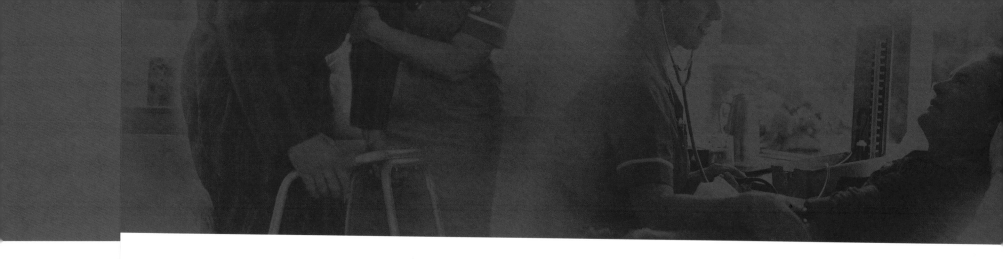

speaking are[...]
indigent em[...]
their privacy [...]
NWRO's law[...]
ten recomm[...]

Not surp[...]
expand its b[...]
consumer or[...]
eral recomm[...]
significantly[...]
amble, which[...]
rights." It de[...]
"equitable a[...]
under all cir[...]
on, "entails a[...]
involved in t[...]
to respect hi[...]
that "no per[...]
treatment or[...]
and medical[...]
erations as r[...]
nature of th[...]
was the first[...]
discriminati[...]
patients on [...]

The prea[...]
tals, a patien[...]
that the pati[...]

suitability to the modern state of the art and to simplify and clarify the language of the standards and interpretations to remove all possible ambiguities and misunderstandings."

With the objective of formulating "optimum achievable" standards, the Joint Commission applied for and received financial assistance from the W. K. Kellogg Foundation. It soon received the first of what would be several large grants from Kellogg that underwrote most of the costs of standards revision. In 1967, after the standards revision process had begun, the Joint Commission was strongly criticized by the Health Benefits Advisory Council, a prestigious advisory group to Medicare. This group said that standards were poorly applied by individual surveyors and that existing standards were inadequate on health and safety conditions in hospitals. The council called for new federal standards, which could in effect mean that the Joint Commission had no role, at least with respect to Medicare. "In response to this criticism," Porterfield later told a reporter, "JCAH introduced team surveys and reduced the maximum interval between surveys from three years to two years." The teams were comprised of a physician and, for the first time, a nurse or administrator. The introduction of teams and the shortening of the survey cycle caused a growth in staff and a rise in fees in the early 1970s.

In view of questioning of its raison d'être, the Joint Commission could certainly not retreat. "What began in 1966 as a fairly simple literary face-lifting of hospital accreditation standards, thought to be a six- to twelve-month operation, has become Project One, the long-promised and impatiently awaited complete revision of the hospital accreditation code for the supportive elements of quality hospital care," Porterfield wrote in the October 1968 *Bulletin*. It was a major undertaking, substantively and organizationally. At its head was Walter W. Carroll, a Chicago surgeon in private practice who was forced to reduce his practice because of arthritis. Carroll, a clinical professor at Northwestern, had recently been president of the Western Surgical Association. At the Joint Commission, his staff included a nurse, a hospital administrator, and a writer.

There were 21 advisory panels consisting of from six to twenty specialists in various fields, including nursing, dietetics, anesthesia, pharmacy, radiology, and fire safety. In the course of the project, 320 experts were reimbursed for expenses and received honoraria for their services. The board's Standards and Survey Procedures Committees reviewed preliminary drafts at intensive one- or two-day meetings. (Survey Procedures, which had been an ad hoc committee, became a standing committee of the board in 1967.) At these meetings, staff proposals were often substantially

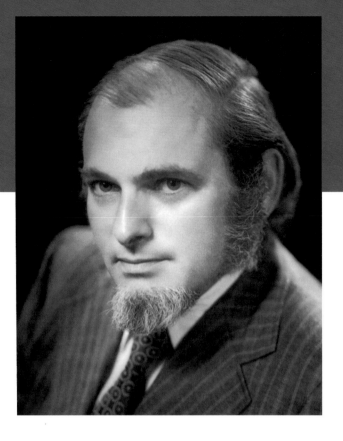

Foundation supported a series of Joint Commission workshops for medical and hospital staff about the standards and their application. State hospital and medical associations cosponsored most of these workshops. They were well attended and well received in the field. Porterfield was pleased to report to the board in April 1972 that nearly 20 percent of attendees were physicians and 5 percent were trustees.

"We hope," Porterfield noted in the *Bulletin* when the latter Kellogg grant was received, "that this educational program will interest state hospital associations and medical societies in cooperating in the development of quality control programs to assist hospitals within the framework of the Joint Commission's evaluation of the total patient-care environment." In 1970, Porterfield had hired Charles M. Jacobs, a bright young lawyer who had previously

been running seminars around the country on hospital law, to run educational programs for the Joint Commission. Jacobs taught workshops and institutes about medical audits and quality control, and developed medical by-laws to meet requirements that courts were beginning to place on hospital boards and medical staffs. The popularity of these educational workshops and institutes allowed the Joint Commission to begin charging for them. The educational programs that Jacobs ran were expected to generate 6.6 percent of the Joint Commission's total budget in 1973.

Also, in 1971, Porterfield made Reed M. Nesbit associate director. Nesbit had been a commissioner from the ACS for 10 years, and he had just completed a term as chairman of the board when he went to work for the Joint Commission full-time. Nesbit was a very prominent, academically based urologist. As a result of a stroke, he could no longer perform surgery, but he remained a forceful personality. Coming from the public health field, Porterfield apparently realized that he needed a strong clinician with an independent power base at his side to help stand up to the clinical organizations. Nesbit and Porterfield formed an effective team.

Computers, which were first used by the Joint Commission during research on standards revision, were soon being used to store data from surveys.

Survey reports and computerized records were kept under lock and key. Not even Porterfield could take records out of the secure room where they were stored. There was great sensitivity at the Joint Commission about confidentiality. It was thought that hospitals would not disclose information about problems if they thought it could be made public or could be subpoenaed by legislatures or subject to discovery in litigation. Others, however, believed that hospitals hid damaging information from the Joint Commission anyway to gain certification. Hospital and medical staffs sometimes privately acknowledged that in addition to sprucing up their institutions prior to a survey, certain records were put in places where they could not be seen.

In 1970, in response to the more demanding consumer environment, the Joint Commission had established a Consumer Advisory Committee, comprised of representatives of 19 consumer organizations. However, this committee spun off by the following year to become the independent National Consumer Coalition on Health Care, with a mission that went beyond advising the Joint Commission. In fact, this coalition soon faulted the Joint Commission for conflict of interest due to "provider domination" and labeled its component organizations "lobbyists for the providers." In the late 1960s and early 1970s, in an effort to enhance popular understanding of its

mission and operations, the Joint Commission's staff sought new opportunities to get its story before the public. They had limited success, but they obviously could not prevent the Joint Commission from being criticized in print, as when it was called the "hired hand" of hospitals or referred to as an "elite," "private," "secretive" organization, accountable to its corporate parents, not to the public. It was understandably painful to the staff and board of commissioners to have their integrity impugned.

In 1970, the constitutionality of the Joint Commission's role as defined by the Medicare Act was challenged in federal district court in Washington, D.C. Five groups of elderly citizens from Washington, D.C., and San Francisco, represented by legal assistance lawyers, cited inadequate conditions and unsafe treatment at D.C. General Hospital and San Francisco General Hospital, both of which were accredited. The plaintiffs alleged that Congress had acted unconstitutionally by relinquishing public authority to a private agency. Since Joint Commission proceedings were secret and not subject to HEW oversight or judicial review, the plaintiffs alleged, they had been denied due process under the Constitution.

While briefs were being prepared and filed in this lawsuit, Congress was considering health care issues and possible legislation. The escalating costs of health care; growing concerns about quality; and inequities, inefficiencies and gaps in the provision of services were all attracting attention in the early 1970s. Naturally, the Joint Commission became part of these discussions in Congress. Some Democratic and Republican legislators wanted the federal government to regulate hospitals directly or through a new council or commission and were ready to scrap voluntary accreditation altogether.

The Joint Commission sometimes seemed exasperated with unrealistic expectations and the questioning of voluntary standards that was occurring in these years. "Consumers and government want much more from us than we are prepared to give," Porterfield told *Hospital Practice* in 1973. The Joint Commission surveyed the "nest," he explained. Accreditation meant that there was a significant likelihood that the "egg" of patient care was not in bad odor and that was about as much as the Joint Commission could realistically do. In 1972, Porterfield testified before the Senate that accreditation "was never intended as a device to protect the public, even though in former decades it was almost the only identifiable benchmark of reliability." "All we can say, with our accreditation," he told Senator Edward M. Kennedy, "[is] that the hospital is apparently living up to normal, reasonably close approximation to nationally adopted standards and that we

have no reason to think that [it] will willfully be in default on a certain day."

"Why is it so important that JCAH should endure?" Carl Schlicke asked the Western Surgical Association in his presidential address in 1972. "If the concept of self-regulation is untenable," he answered portentously, "the very concept of self-government is at stake."

Senator Abraham Ribicoff of Connecticut, a former HEW secretary, led a bipartisan majority toward strengthening government oversight without abandoning voluntary accreditation. In the Ribicoff amendments to the Medicare Act in 1972, Congress gave the secretary of HEW authority to carry out validation surveys of Joint Commission-accredited hospitals participating in Medicare. HEW was similarly authorized to conduct surveys of accredited hospitals on the basis of complaints alleging noncompliance with Medicare standards and was authorized to establish standards that exceeded the Joint Commission's. These amendments mooted the pending lawsuits, while also meaning that the relationship between the Joint Commission and government would necessarily become closer.

MANIFESTATIONS OF GROWTH

The growth in the Joint Commission's scope and scale, just from 1969 to 1973, is reflected in its budget.

In 1972, *the bimonthly* Perspectives on Accreditation *replaced the* Bulletin.

A memorandum prepared for the Executive Committee in March 1973 reported that total income had increased from $1.3 million in 1969 to a projected $4.5 million in 1973, very nearly a 250 percent increase. The largest dollar growth was in survey fees, which accounted for 51.5 percent of income in 1969 and 70.2 percent in 1973. Contributions from corporate and council members had increased 23.2 percent but these contributions represented a diminishing percentage of total income, down to 8.7 percent from 23.2 percent in 1969.

Although inflation contributed significantly to increases in both costs and income in these years, the biggest factor was simply growth in the number of personnel, which occurred in the new and old programs alike and in central administration. At the end of 1969, the Joint Commission had approximately 65 employees and at the end of 1972, it had 170 employees. Salaries increased from $652,000 to $2.25 million over five years. Fringe benefits and travel and maintenance followed the trend in salaries. Expenses for the hospital accreditation program, which was the largest, increased three-fold as a result of changes that had been made in the frequency and procedures of surveys and inflation.

The Joint Commission's expansion brought a change in its newsletter. The *Bulletin* had in recent years been a quarterly, devoted mainly to Joint Commission policy and distributed to hospitals and their medical staffs. It was replaced by *Perspectives on Accreditation* in January 1972, which was published bimonthly and distributed to the combined mailing lists of the Joint Commission's various programs. It contained information about specific programs as well as more general subjects. Inserts

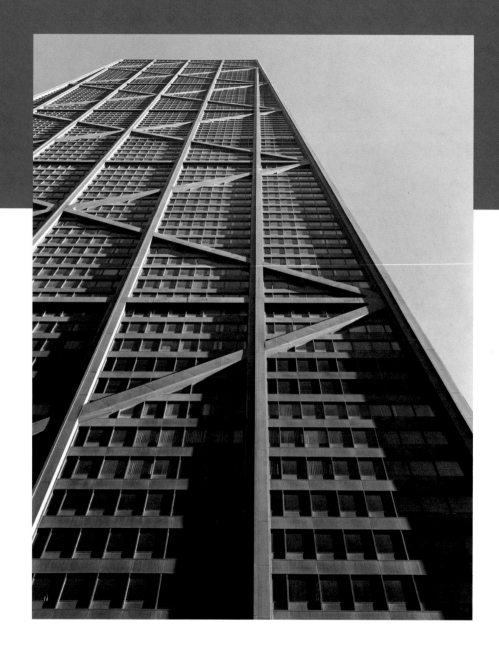

▲ ▶ *Having outgrown the offices at the Blair Building due to continuing program expansion, the Joint Commission moved its headquarters to the John Hancock building in 1973, above and opposite. The organization occupied the 22nd floor of the towering Chicago landmark.*

targeted to particular audiences could also be included in the mailing.

With its lease at the Blair Building set to expire in April 1973, the Joint Commission began to look for new offices a year in advance. It wanted more space and a more efficient layout. In early 1973, the Joint Commission moved to the 22nd floor of the towering John Hancock building at 875 North Michigan Avenue. The board convened there for the first time in April. But it returned to the Lake Shore Club in August for a special two-day "think tank" session with additional invited guests from corporate and council members.

There was no doubt that much had changed in recent years. After defending its purpose and methods to numerous detractors and after instituting dramatic changes to accommodate explosive growth, the Joint Commission was rewarded with new organizational challenges and stresses. But in recognition of the constancy of such challenges, the board sat to consider the Joint Commission's long range philosophy and plans in structure, standards, research, education, and hospital-doctor relations.

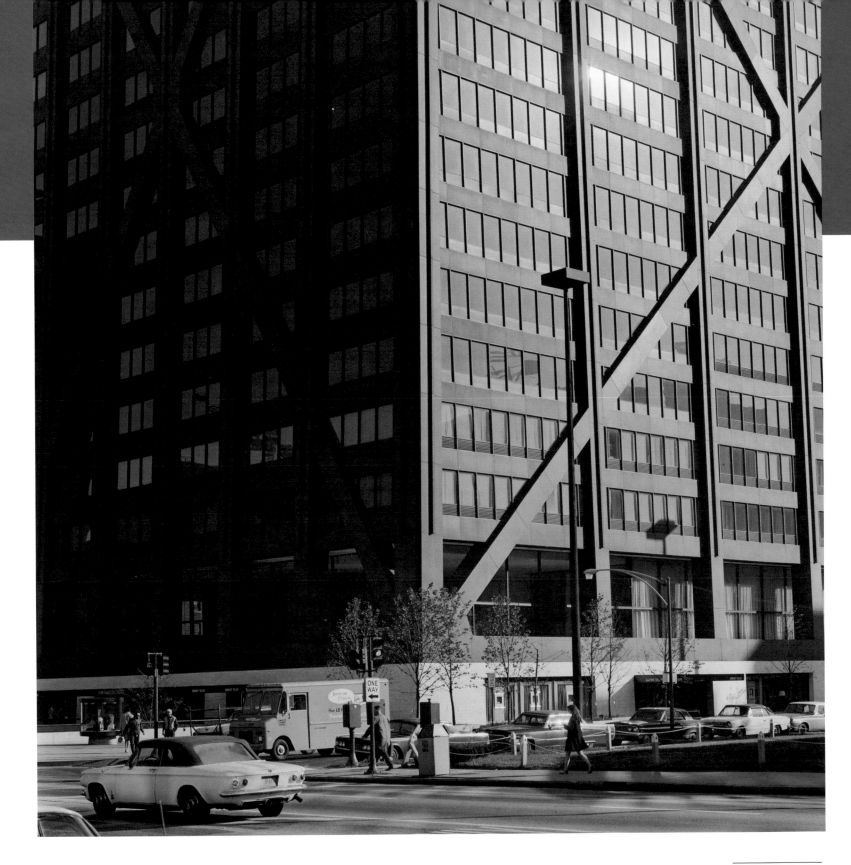

From Reorganization to an Agenda for Change

On December 17, 1976, the Joint Commission celebrated its 25th anniversary with a formal dinner at Chez Paul in Chicago. It was an evening for toasts and nostalgia held in the very building that originally served as the Joint Commission's headquarters. Kenneth Babcock and John Porterfield traced the Joint Commission's history for the assembled guests, who included current commissioners; former chairmen of the board, accreditation council chairmen and program directors; and the CEOs of the four member organizations.

Marjorie Lynch, undersecretary of the Department of Health, Education and Welfare (HEW) and the featured speaker that evening, focused on the relationship between the Joint Commission and the federal government since the enactment of Medicare in 1965. "We were grateful that there was a Joint Commission when the Medicare legislation was passed," she said. "If there had not been one, we would have had to establish one, since the hospital certification require-

ments mandated by Congress could not have been satisfied in any other way."

Lynch observed that the 1972 amendments to the Social Security Act had dramatically affected the relationship between the government and the Joint Commission. These amendments had authorized validation surveys as well as the creation of Professional Standards Review Organizations, both of which overlapped with the activities of the Joint Commission. In 1973, Congress also had nurtured the growth of Health Maintenance Organizations (HMOs) by mandating that employers of 25 or more persons who offered health insurance to their employees offer them the option of joining a qualified HMO if one existed in their area. HMOs appealed to public officials, including key members of the Nixon administration, because of HMOs' emphasis on preventive health care and the promise of lower costs.

Health care providers were having to deal with an expanding regulatory environment at both the federal

Although the Joint Commission had accomplished a great deal during its first 25 years, it was on shaky ground in 1976.

and state levels. In fact, increasing government regulation merely reflected crosscurrents in public opinion — an almost insatiable demand for more and better health care services coupled with concerns about rising costs and who was to pay for them. These crosscurrents are still swirling today, but in the mid-1970s, it appeared to many that it was only a matter of time before national health insurance was a reality. While the government sought to reduce costs through more efficient utilization of facilities and services, federal- and state-supported programs in professional education, training and scientific research were simultaneously driving up the demand for upgraded facilities and services. Each new technology, test, or medical specialty that resulted from these programs contributed to the increasing cost of health care.

Reflecting on the more than 11 years since the passage of Medicare, Lynch concluded, "our collaborative relationship could serve as a model in the health care field for relations between government and the voluntary sector." Indeed, the message reinforced the statements of Theodore Cooper, assistant secretary of HEW and a physician, who the previous August had also spoken to the board of commissioners. Cooper addressed mounting concerns about HEW's reports to Congress, which contained some criticisms directed at the Joint Commission. "It would be a great loss if, due to our activity, you concluded that your role is no longer necessary," Cooper said. "To us, the JCAH is a necessary part of American medicine."

But by the anniversary dinner in December, Lynch and Cooper, appointees of President Gerald R. Ford, who was defeated in November by Governor Jimmy Carter of Georgia, were lame ducks. Although the Joint Commission had accomplished a great deal during its first 25 years, it was on shaky ground in 1976. John Westerman, who joined the board that year as an AHA representative, recalls a constant feeling of crisis at the time over the Joint Commission's mission, objectives, and organization. The board's Planning and Organization Committee, under Carl P. Schlicke's chairmanship, had spent much of the year leading up to the anniversary reflecting, with the assistance of staff, on where the Joint Commission had been, assessing its current status and contemplating its future. The exercise had resulted in the board's determination that the best course was "to continue its combined focus on the quality of health-related care, in its broadest definition, working with the professional providers of care to maintain and improve that quality."

With funding from foundation grants, the Joint Commission had in 1975 established its newest accreditation council — the Council for Ambulatory Health Care — to accredit facilities in the burgeoning field of non-hospital health services. There was also a growing trend in these years toward group medical practices

Life safety was the primary reason for hospitals to fail validation surveys. There had been no known multiple-death fire incident in American hospitals since 1954.

as the Joint Commission's weakest spot and to demonstrate the invalidity of JCAH surveys because of that one weakness."

By 1975, 105 hospitals had lost their "deemed status" as a result of these inspections. Two-thirds of the rejections involved life safety issues exclusively or in conjunction with some other area of physical plant deficiency. The Joint Commission actually liberalized its more tolerant policy on deficiencies in 1975, giving hospitals two years, rather than one, to make what were often expensive capital improvements in the area of building safety. Not surprisingly, accredited hospitals that lost their "deemed status" complained to the Joint Commission, but the Bureau of Health Insurance disregarded the Joint Commission's objections to the conduct of the validation surveys and denied it any channel through which to appeal validation decisions.

Life safety was the primary reason for hospitals to fail validation surveys. There had been no known multiple-death fire incident in American hospitals since 1954, though there had been single deaths by fires. Their causes did not relate primarily to structural defects, and were often smoking-related. But with the federal government raising the bar on fire safety and building codes, the Joint Commission quickly set to work strengthening its own standards, hiring additional staff with expertise in this area, to preserve the link between accreditation and "deemed

and away from individual practices. Specialization and sub-specialization also were expanding.

Government's greater regulatory role in health care certainly did affect the Joint Commission. In 1973 and 1974, validation teams were sent out by the states, under the auspices of the Bureau of Health Insurance in the Social Security Administration. The state teams, primarily engineers and fire safety experts, as opposed to health professionals, were strictly inspectional, offering no consultation and heavily emphasizing physical plant, building codes and fire safety. The Joint Commission survey, on the other hand, relied upon the most recent reports hospitals had received from state licensing agencies and fire marshals with respect to building codes and fire safety. Porterfield told the board that federal and state inspectors were "apparently determined to concentrate the validation survey on what they perceive

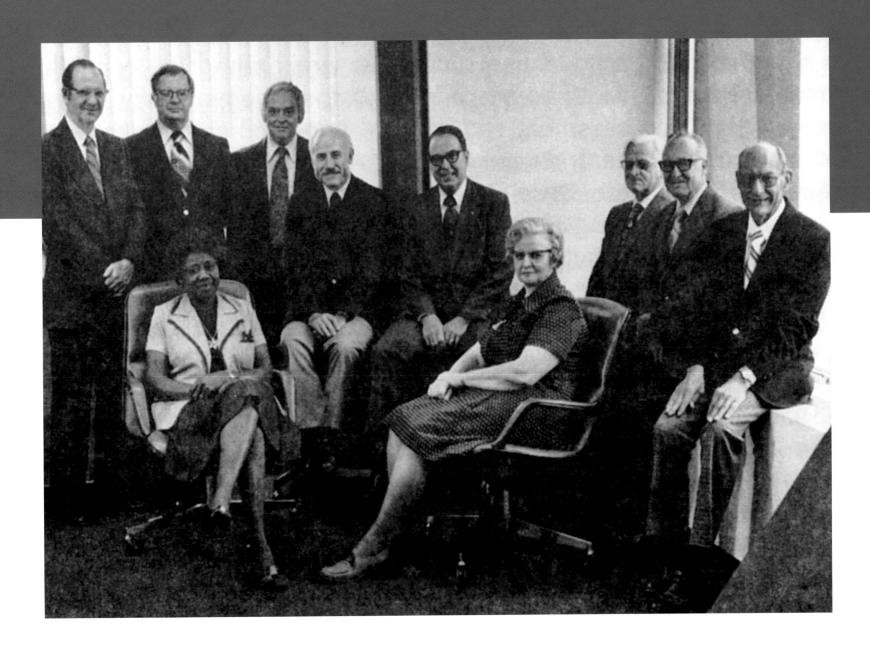

status." This effort continued and expanded through the 1980s, when the Joint Commission developed a professional division dedicated to that area, but the validation surveys had already hurt the Joint Commission's credibility with hospitals and weakened its relationship with government.

Compounding the growing level of distrust was a breach of confidentiality by HEW, to whom the

▲ *Pictured is a hospital surveyor training class in 1975. Since the Stover Committee Report of 1956, the Joint Commission had employed full-time, paid surveyors to conduct the hospital visits. Training of these surveyors has always been a high priority for the commission.*

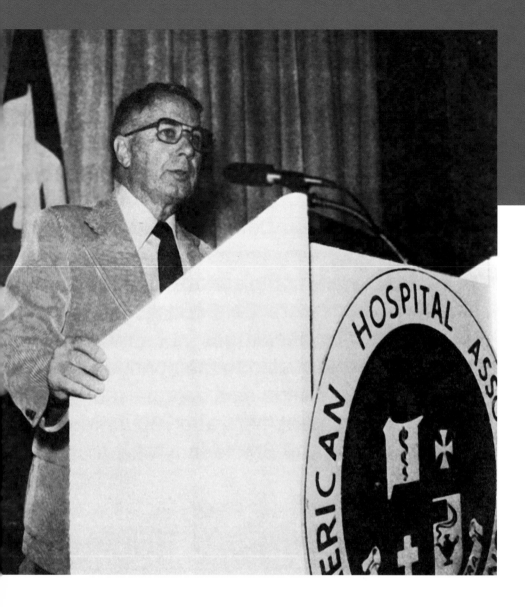

▲ *John E. Affeldt, who like John Porterfield came from the public health field, became president of the Joint Commission in 1977. Here Affeldt addresses the American Hospital Association's annual convention shortly after his appointment.*

Joint Commission had released survey reports on a confidential basis. When a consumer organization brought litigation against HEW, some of the reports were released publicly during the case. In 1975, the Joint Commission itself successfully brought suit against HEW in order to prevent future breaches of confidentiality.

In a presentation to the board in August 1975, Porterfield described the Joint Commission's paradoxical position. On the one hand, the board had taken the position that it should maintain equivalency with government regulations, for example, in securing a clean "deemed status" as allowed by Medicare. On the other hand, professional groups asserted that the Joint Commission was itself beginning to resemble a government agency. Porterfield observed that "what started sixty years ago as a consultative support and improvement program from within the professions is now being proposed as basis for certification (e.g., for reimbursement by Medicare, for licensing by the California Department of Health.)" The Joint Commission had begun to cooperate with the California Medical Association in a program whereby the Joint Commission and the California Department of Health jointly surveyed hospitals. Through this program, accreditation could be tantamount to state licensure, an implication which the board was loath to accept.

The Joint Commission was, in Porterfield's view, endeavoring to do two things that were not completely compatible. It had to decide exactly what its role was and announce that role. This was not merely a philosophical question, he said, for it would affect both standards and survey procedures. The current standards were highly general with long interpretations that allowed professional discretion in particular situations. Those kinds of standards did not work in a certification process, however, which employed literal application of precise regulations. Porterfield called for a clear statement of the Joint Commission's objectives in accreditation.

By the 25th anniversary celebration, Porterfield had informed the board of his intention to retire as director. Although it was his decision to step down, it seems unlikely that the board was distressed to hear that news. Reportedly, some of the corporate and board members felt that Porterfield was spending too much time in California and not enough attending to business in Chicago.

AFFELDT APPOINTMENT

At a special meeting in March 1977, the search committee introduced a candidate for the directorship to the board, a retired general. The last time the board had offered the job to a general, he had withdrawn as a candidate. This time around, the board had reservations, reportedly because of concerns that the candidate might be too rigid, so they asked the search committee to pursue other possibilities. The next month,

Carl Schlicke, who had become chairman of the board, introduced John E. Affeldt to the board as "director-designate."

Affeldt recalls that when a surgeon friend first asked him whether he would be interested in the position, he surprised himself by saying yes, for he had in recent years turned down all other job overtures. He remembers being interviewed in Chicago by Schlicke and the CEOs of the AMA, the AHA, and the ACS: James H. Sammons, J. Alexander McMahon and C. Rollins Hanlon, respectively. One of the key questions he recalls was whether he would live in Chicago. Affeldt answered affirmatively. Indeed, he rented an apartment in an upper floor of the John Hancock Building, so he lived "above the store" throughout his tenure.

At the time of his appointment, Affeldt was medical director of the Los Angeles County Department of Health Services, where he oversaw a large, complex public health system. He was also president of the American Congress of Rehabilitation Medicine, a fellow of the ACP, and a member of the AMA and regional medical societies. Affeldt held faculty appointments at the University of Southern California and the University of California at Los Angeles, and he had served on numerous advisory boards in California and with HEW. He was able, thoughtful, a good public speaker and a man of integrity and decency. Moreover, he possessed good people skills and was at home with bureaucratic processes.

Affeldt had graduated from Andrews University in his home state of Michigan and had gone to medical school at Loma Linda University in Los Angeles. While he was doing a residency in internal medicine, a polio epidemic struck Los Angeles. That led to his involvement in a research study funded by the Polio Foundation and based at Harvard University. In the early 1950s, Affeldt played a major role in establishing a respiratory treatment center for polio victims in Downey, California, that led him into a career as a medical administrator. From 1964 until 1972, he had been the medical director of Los Angeles' municipal hospitals, giving ample evidence of his political and organizational skill. Age 59 when he assumed the directorship, Affeldt was older than his predecessors had been, but he had valuable years of experience and the relaxed confidence to take on the job laid out by Porterfield.

Fully cooperating with Affeldt during the transition, Porterfield was frank about organizational deficiencies. He was also frank in his farewell statement in *Perspectives*. Although voicing no regrets about the expansion of accreditation into new areas, he acknowledged that management had failed to integrate the new programs or to develop shared protocols among them. At the outset, he explained, programs simply tried to establish themselves securely, and, now that they were secure, it would be difficult, though necessary, to integrate them. He disagreed with the assumption that the Joint Commission was now serving as an agent of government but argued that it could play an expanding role as an intermediary between government and providers of care. Although Porterfield did not report this fact to his readership, in December he had given the board his strongly held opinion that the time had come for it to have consumer or public representation.

During the hiring process, the search committee agreed to change the director's title to the currently popular one of president and chief executive officer, a change which was implemented by the board when Affeldt took over from Porterfield in August 1977. At that time, George Graham, who had stepped down as chairman of the Joint Commission in 1976 to become its deputy director, became vice president for external affairs, liaison to HEW and health care organizations. Formerly president of the AHA, Graham had a medical degree and a significant career in hospital administration. At the same time, George Coldewey, who had been with the Joint Commission for three years, was named vice president for operations, charged with consolidating the Joint Commission's operating units. Associate Director Reed Nesbit resigned on account of his deteriorating health, and his position was not filled — probably a mistake, Charles Jacobs later

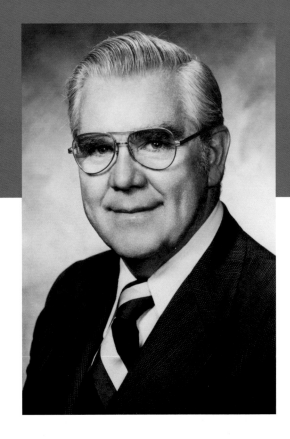

observed, because Nesbit had great stature with the clinical organizations.

In a speech to the AHA convention soon after he became president, Affeldt announced the Joint Commission's objective to study its relationship with the accreditation councils and to formulate a plan for reorganizing its diffuse parts. The principal options under consideration were a federation of accrediting bodies, a consolidation of current accreditation programs, and a return to the original hospital accreditation program, which implied terminating the new programs. Affeldt voiced the most critical question facing the Joint Commission: "Can the voluntary approach to assuring the quality of health care prevail, or will it become a function of government?" In order for the voluntary approach to survive, he cautioned, providers would have to "support and comply with principles, standards, and procedures sufficiently detailed and comprehensive to assure all concerned parties that the optimal achievable level of service is being provided, and that deviations from this level of service are identifiable."

The public, third-party payers, legislators and regulators, in Affeldt's view, "must become and remain convinced that the JCAH, although a creation of health care organizations, is neither a captive nor a tool of those organizations to be used for satisfying their own self-interests." Legislators and the public also needed to be made aware of hazards associated

with the government's becoming the primary purchaser of health services through a national health insurance plan. "If and when this plan becomes a reality," Affeldt cautioned, "the government will become the regulator of both cost and quality, with the added probability that its own interest in cost control would take precedence over considerations regarding quality." Everyone would have to do a much better job of demonstrating that voluntarily determined and enforced standards, currently at risk, best served the public interest.

REORGANIZATION AND PTACs

By 1977, thanks in part to the groundwork laid by the Planning and Organization Committee, the board had reached a consensus that the council structure was dysfunctional. Within the board, and especially among AHA commissioners, there were always some

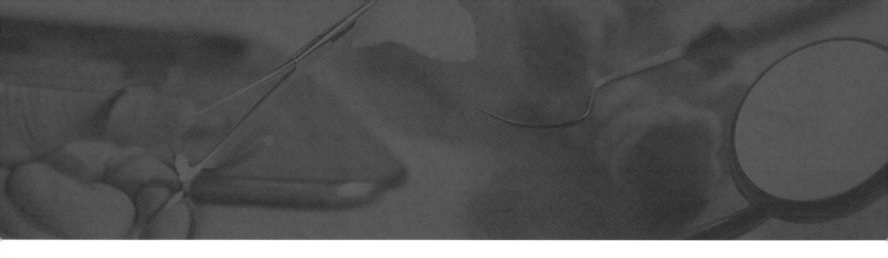

doubts about non-hospital programs. The accreditation councils were seen as too autonomous and as unresponsive to the commission as a whole. They controlled their own budgets, determined their own fees, hired their own staffs and set their own standards and survey procedures. There was somewhat of a culture gap between the commission and the councils as well. Typically, the councils were comprised of younger men and women, in contrast to the older and predominantly male board of commissioners. Council members were often "hot-shots in their fields," John Westerman recalls, and were disdainful of "clubby, cigar-smoking board members," whom they saw as being in the twilight of their careers, though Westerman himself, only 43 years old when he joined the board, negated that assumption. Affeldt was charged with reorganizing the structure, and the corporate members assessed themselves $30,000 per seat or $600,000 in total to cover the costs of reorganization.

Paul Sanazaro, a physician, had recently run an HEW division that was concerned with quality assurance, and he was known as a pioneer in that area. Affeldt, in agreement with most of Sanazaro's ideas, hired him as a consultant to work closely with the Planning and Organization Committee (now chaired by John Graham) and with Affeldt and other staff members. According to Affeldt, it was Sanazaro who was the principal author of the reorganization plan.

At a special meeting on October 28, 1978, the board, which was now chaired by Schlicke, instituted the plan by voting to do the following:

1. To terminate the Memoranda of Agreement establishing the four accreditation councils, effective no later than June 30, 1979.

2. To establish a Policy Advisory Committee of not more than 30 individuals to provide policy advice to the board of commissioners and also serve as a forum for the exchange of information regarding national and professional issues affecting the Joint Commission and its voluntary accreditation role.

3. To establish Professional and Technical Advisory Committees (PTACs) to provide professional and technical advice to each of the relevant programs. (In addition to the four programs that had accreditation councils, there would be a separate PTAC for the hospital program.)

4. To endorse the president's managerial plans, including the establishment of a division of accreditation, a division of education and publications, and a department of corporate planning. (Donald C. Smith, who had recently been a professor of pediatrics and maternal and child health at the University of Michigan, was soon named vice president, in charge of the new division of accreditation.)

The board that day also approved initiation of a study on long-range planning, including an examination of its own composition. Among the items to be

This reorganization was hardly embraced by the councils, which viewed it with varying degrees of hope, anxiety, and revulsion.

considered was a revision of the Joint Commission's mission and scope statement, long-range policy toward national health care interests, and relations with state and federal government.

This reorganization was hardly embraced by the councils, which viewed it with varying degrees of hope, anxiety, and revulsion. Even though council members would be eligible to become PTAC members, that determination would be made by the Joint Commission, which would also exercise much greater control over individual programs than it had previously exercised. Following negotiations and deliberations, two of the councils, the Accreditation Council for Psychiatric Facilities and the Accreditation Council for Long Term Care, went along with the new order of things. Staff members with those two councils moved over to become program directors at the Joint Commission, Elaine Nelson in long-term care and Myrene McAninch in psychiatric facilities, respectively.

The nascent Council for Ambulatory Health Care, however, was sharply divided, with some members, particularly those from the older clinical organizations, wanting to remain under the Joint Commission umbrella, and other members, especially those from group medical organizations, not wishing to do so. Indeed, the latter group split off to form the Accreditation Association for Ambulatory Health Care. It became and has remained a major competitor

to the Joint Commission's surviving ambulatory care program, which was directed by Elizabeth Flanagan. The Accreditation Council for Services for the Mentally Retarded and Other Developmentally Disabled Persons also left the Joint Commission in 1979. The Joint Commission remained in this field, however, through its surveys of community mental health centers under its program in psychiatry.

"It was a power struggle at base," summarizes John Milton, a veteran staff member in the hospital program, "with a lot of blood on the floor." But in the long run, the PTACs strengthened the role of a wide range of health care organizations in standard-setting, which was one of their primary objectives. At the same time, they allowed the Joint Commission to become a stronger and more cohesive organization, enhancing its legitimacy, effectiveness, and acceptance among health care professionals and providers alike.

In the fall and winter of 1979, with assistance from consultants Jacques Cousin and William Fifer, the board turned to the second phase of the reorganization. At the conclusion of this process, the board reaffirmed its basic philosophy of accreditation, which it defined as "a voluntary and professional activity that strives, by means of consultation and education, to enable health care facilities and programs to provide the optimal achievable quality of patient care." It also initiated changes in board composition. It rejected reducing the number of AMA and AHA seats and turning them over to other organizations, but it unanimously agreed to give a seat to the American Dental Association (ADA). The board also took Porterfield's suggestion to add a public representative, contingent on the establishment of criteria for membership, a selection process and a method of financing the seat. (Ultimately the Joint Commission itself absorbed the costs, which was the only thing it could do.)

Many dentists, including oral and maxillofacial surgeons, as well as general and pediatric dentists, cared for patients in acute care hospitals and other institutions that the Joint Commission accredited, including specialty hospitals and nursing homes. Dentists, who constituted the second-largest group of health professionals with doctoral degrees, had distinct needs and expertise. The ADA had of course long sought to become a member of the Joint Commission, but had repeatedly been turned down. Through the years, controversies, both nationally and locally, had raged over staff privileges for dentists. In 1979, however, the ADA had let it be known that it was prepared to sue to become a member. The Joint Commission was already a defendant in other antitrust lawsuits, as will be seen, and there was no interest in defending another one.

Affeldt recalls an informal conversation with McMahon, Sammons, and Hanlon in which it was agreed that if the ADA were to sue, they would not defend the case. Rather than leave the decision to the mercy of the courts, they decided to offer the ADA one seat, rather than the two seats it was seeking. The ADA accepted the Joint Commission's invitation in December 1979, and the corporate by-laws were amended accordingly. "The Board's decision to expand its corporate membership is a milestone in the history of JCAH," Affeldt observed in *Perspectives*.

The American Nurses' Association (ANA), the largest nursing organization, like the ADA, had in the past requested a seat on the Joint Commission's board. But as it happened, ANA was experiencing financial difficulties and was in no position to pay corporate dues or to begin legal action to claim a board seat. Instead of offering board representation, the Joint Commission asked both the ANA and the Association of Operating Room Nurses to appoint representatives to the newly created hospital PTAC. ANA and the National League for Nursing also served on the newly formed Policy Advisory Committee. The AHA also agreed to select one of its own representatives on the board of commissioners from the American Organization of Nurse Executives, with which it was affiliated. This representation was well deserved. Not only did nurses constitute the largest number of health care professionals, but also approximately 90 of the Joint Commission's 300 employees were RNs, who served the organization as surveyors, counselors, consultants and educators, as Affeldt pointed out at the ANA's June 1978 convention in Hawaii. And that same year, when the hospital nursing standards were under revision, 20 national leaders in nursing were invited to the Joint Commission's headquarters for discussion of current issues in nursing. Subsequently, 600 copies of the first draft of the nursing standards were distributed to organizations and individuals for comment.

Thus at the board's first meeting in 1980, Charles A. "Scotty" McCallum and Barbara Donaho took their places at the table as representatives from the ADA and the AHA, respectively. Donaho was vice president and director of nursing at a Minneapolis hospital, and she soon became corporate director of nursing for the Sisters of Mercy Health Corporation in Farmington Hills, Michigan. She was a former president and board member of the American Society of Nursing Service Administrators. At the time of her appointment, she was chairman of the AHA Council on Nursing.

During her seven very active years on the board of commissioners, Donaho served on and then chaired the Accreditation Committee, one of the key standing committees. In that position, she oversaw a shift to more open, systematic and quantitative processes of accreditation as well as faster reports to the field. It should be noted that nurses had previously served on the board of commissioners, though they were nurses who became hospital administrators.

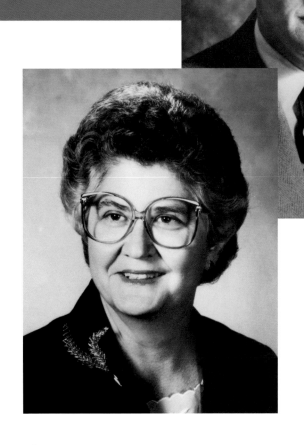

▲ *Charles A. "Scotty" McCallum and Barbara Donaho both joined the board of commissioners in 1980. McCallum, the first representative from the American Dental Association, chaired the board in 1987 and 1988. In response to pressure from the nursing profession for a seat on the board, the American Hospital Association agreed to select one of its own representatives from the American Organization of Nurse Executives. The first such representative was Donaho, who went on to chair the Joint Commission's accreditation committee.*

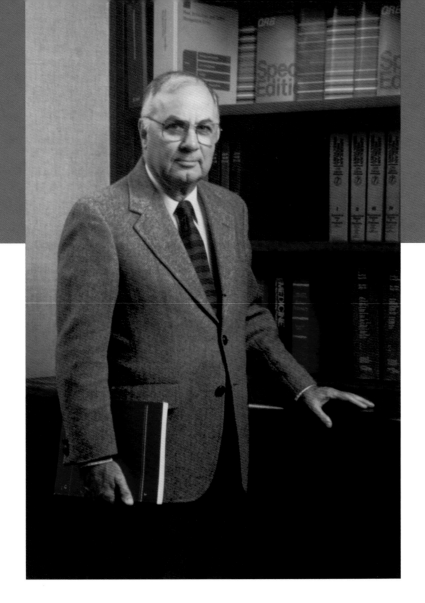

Medical Center at the University of Alabama in Birmingham. When McCallum first joined the board, it was undecided whether the ADA would become part of the traditional rotation of officers, including the chairmanship. But McCallum so impressed his fellow commissioners in his first two years that he was made an officer without controversy. That put him in line to chair the board, which he did in 1987 and 1988. Since every organization was represented on each of the Joint Commission's standing committees, McCallum, who was the only ADA member, felt obliged to serve on each of them, and this made his burden particularly heavy. In the late 1980s, McCallum spent 50 to 60 days a year at meetings in Chicago.

After the ADA had been admitted to Joint Commission corporate membership, the board changed the medical staff by-law standards to enable "qualified dental surgeons to perform history and physical examinations on their own patients admitted for dental surgery" at hospitals, although many doctors worried that this would open the question of staff privileges for other non-medical practitioners. In 1982, the ADA's accreditation program for hospital dental services was incorporated into the Joint Commission's hospital accreditation program, and the ADA soon began to participate in surveyor training.

William G. Mitchell, a Chicago lawyer and businessman, who was president of Central Telephone and Utilities Corporation, became the first public

McCallum, an oral surgeon, was an appropriate pioneer representative from the ADA, as he also held a medical degree. (Ironically, some people at the ADA were wary of McCallum, he recalls, *because* he had a medical degree.) But all members of the board were impressed with his distinguished background and, when they got to know him, with his great abilities and personal qualities. McCallum had been dean of the dental school at the University of Alabama in Birmingham from 1962 until 1977. At the time of his appointment to the Joint Commission, he was vice president for health affairs and director of the

member of the board in 1982, probably a frustrating experience. He was succeeded three years later by William G. Beers, the retired chairman and chief executive officer of Kraft, Inc. Although there was only so much that a single public representative could accomplish on what had become a 22-member board, Beers made a valiant effort. He was unintimidated by the steady diet of technical questions and by the professional backgrounds of his fellow commissioners. Beers served on the Accreditation Committee and took to heart his responsibility to represent the public. As Donald Avant, who directed the hospital accreditation program explains, if a hospital failed a survey, "that was it, that didn't fly." Beers, he recalls, "came down on the hospital like 10 tons of bricks."

ADMINISTRATIVE CHANGES AND A MORE ASSERTIVE BOARD

Along with more inclusive representation, Affeldt sought to improve communications and foster cooperation with the Joint Commission's multiple constituencies, including hospitals, professional organizations, government, and the public. Aiding him were several new staff members. Affeldt named Paul E. Mullen director of a new government relations office in 1978. A hospital administrator by training, Mullen had in recent years worked in the AHA's office in Washington, primarily in the area of Medicare institutional standards. Mullen was based in Chicago, where

he covered both federal and state relations and traveled as necessary. In 1980, Affeldt hired Donald W. Avant as director of the hospital accreditation program. Avant had 26 years of experience in hospital administration and public health in Los Angeles, where he became a friend and colleague of Affeldt. At the time of his appointment at the Joint Commission, Avant was chief executive officer of a general hospital in Alameda County, California. Within several years, Affeldt asked Avant to oversee operations in all accreditation programs, at which point, John Milton, who had helped manage the hospital accreditation program since 1976, became its director.

In 1979, Affeldt named James S. Roberts assistant vice president for accreditation. For the previous three years, Roberts, an internist, had been medical director of a multi-specialty group practice in Rochester, New York. From 1971 to 1976, Roberts had worked at HEW, in quality assurance, peer review and research. In his new position at the Joint Commission, Roberts began by trying to strengthen the ambulatory health program and develop long-range planning options for the division of accreditation. He was quickly engaged in improving surveyor education and performance and in formulating new quality assurance standards and procedures. When Don Smith resigned in 1981, Affeldt named Roberts to succeed him as vice president for accreditation. Following George Graham's retirement in 1982, Lawrence A. Hill, a hospital

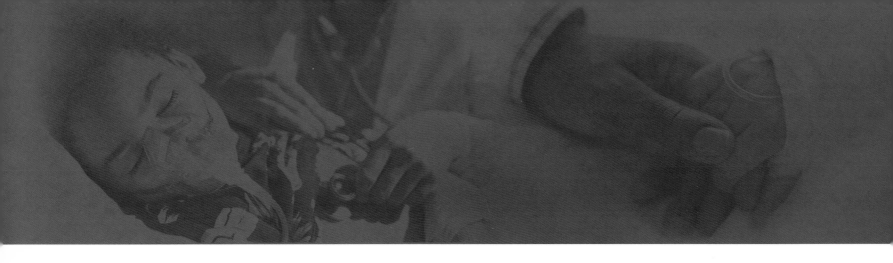

administrator and former executive vice president of the AHA, became vice president for administration.

The reduction of duplicative accreditation activities was one of Affeldt's primary goals. In 1978, the Joint Commission began to cooperate with the College of American Pathologists in the accreditation of hospital laboratories. In California, the Joint Commission surveyed hospitals simultaneously with state licensing or certification teams, which reduced interruptions to normal hospital operations. In three states, the Joint Commission enjoyed deemed status, that is, if a hospital were accredited, the hospital would also be licensed. In a growing number of states, accreditation was under consideration for the purposes of full or partial licensure. The ambiguity of the Joint Commission's position, as observed by Porterfield in 1975, was still evident. However, the sands were shifting toward the Joint Commission accepting a more regulatory role.

In 1979, the U.S. General Accounting Office released a report, two years in the making, that constituted an endorsement of the Joint Commission. GAO compared the system of hospital accreditation for Medicare purposes administered by HEW with the Joint Commission's accreditation decision and survey process. The report's conclusion was that "the JCAH process achieves more consistent results because a single accreditation committee determines compliance based on the independent recommenda-

tions of surveyors, report reviewers and senior program managers." By contrast, there were considerable regional variations in HEW's program. GAO also found that the Joint Commission program was significantly more economical than HEW's. It even suggested that Congress contract with the Joint Commission to conduct all certification surveys. That did not happen, but the worry of several years earlier about the Joint Commission losing deemed status was lessened. In 1980, another GAO report praised the cooperative arrangements the Joint Commission had made with several states for a single survey for both licensure and accreditation purposes. GAO encouraged the expansion of such arrangements.

The Joint Commission expanded its educational activities during this period as well. For most of the Affeldt years, these programs were directed by E. Martin Egelston, who had come from the AHA, while publications were directed by Maryanne Shanahan. Educational programs and publications combined to provide 23 percent of revenues in 1980 and 19 percent in 1981. In 1974, the Joint Commission had begun to publish the *Quality Review Bulletin*. By the early 1980s, it was publishing 12 issues a year, offering practical assistance on quality assurance activities and patient care evaluation techniques. It was designed to meet the needs of a variety of staff members in the field, and it included many special edi-

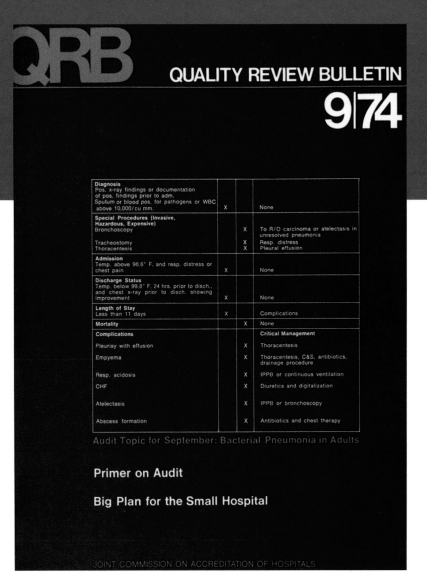

▶ *The* Quality Review Bulletin, *which has been published by the Joint Commission since 1974, offers practical assistance on quality assurance activities and patient care evaluation techniques.*

tions on particular topics. *Perspectives*, manuals, and audiocassettes and videocassette were also steady sellers in these years. The Quality Resource Center, which had also been started under Porterfield and which was directed after 1978 by Egelston, offered a growing number of educational seminars, workshops, and clinics in the 1980s. In 1980, the Joint Commission established a 24-hour hotline to respond to urgent questions and problems from health care organizations and professionals.

The bulk of the Joint Commission's income (76 percent in 1980, 79 percent in 1981) still derived from survey fees, however. Inflationary pressure forced it to raise these fees for all its programs except psychiatric facilities. (It had a different rate structure in mental health because its surveys were generally shorter than those of acute care hospitals.) As of January 1, 1980, fees for the hospital and ambulatory health programs were raised 10 percent to $600 per surveyor day. Fees for the long-term program increased to $500 per surveyor day. These fees were increased by $25 per surveyor day in 1981. In 1982, it was announced, the hospital rate would be hiked all the way to $1,000 per surveyor day.

Though the Joint Commission's accreditation program had been judged efficient by the federal government, in the field, there was unhappiness over rising fees, continuous revision in standards, new program staff in Chicago and the reorganization

itself. There also seemed to be more than the usual number of complaints about uneven performance by surveyors. It seemed everybody had something bad to say about surveyors. Although the board's own Accreditation Committee, not field surveyors, made accreditation decisions, surveyors were the face of the Joint Commission in the field. Affeldt and Roberts were endeavoring to address surveyor problems through improved training, more selective recruitment, and higher salaries. In response to criticisms that physician surveyors were too old, they lowered the average age from 62 in 1977 to 58 by 1981, but much remained to be done to satisfy the various complaints from the field.

And resistance to change was not coming just from the field. In fact, in response to complaints about rising survey fees, the Planning and Organization Committee had been striving to make the corporation more manageable, encouraging financial planning, the establishment of a reserve fund and increased grant-procurement and fundraising. Though sound ideas on the surface, these measures, if implemented, would make the Joint Commission more autonomous and less dependent on its corporate parents, a possibility that sparked concern at the AHA and the AMA, who relished the leverage their financial support of the organization gave them. (In past practice, it was suggested, some AHA and AMA members had used budgetary concerns to purge a staff member or a program of which they did not approve.)

The Planning and Organization Committee was protected by the mandate of the board, but Affeldt, the most visible agent of the committee, was an exposed target. At the end of 1980, Daniel Ellis, who was about to assume the board chairmanship, heard that Alex McMahon and Jim Sammons, the CEOs of the AHA and the AMA respectively, were conspiring to remove Affeldt. Scotty McCallum urged Ellis to

call a meeting and resolve the issue. The off-the-record meeting convened at the O'Hare Hilton on a frigid day in early 1981. The CEOs of the original parent organizations were present, as were many commissioners, but Affeldt was not invited.

It was appropriate that Ellis chaired the meeting. Prior to his appointment to the board, he had been a regent of the ACP, where he had no contact with the Joint Commission, though he had heard many complaints about its surveying process at ACP regents meetings and at Massachusetts General Hospital, where he was a longtime staff member. Ellis was the director of quality assurance at MGH and was known as the hospital's "conscience."

Though he was not directly involved, Ellis's opinions paralleled the objectives of the reorganization of the late 1970s. As a regent, Ellis had voted against contributing additional funds to the Joint Commission to support its expansion into ambulatory care. Ellis felt that the Joint Commission should not expand until it did a better job with hospitals. He was in the minority on the ACP board of regents on that issue, but in 1975 he was asked to serve on the board of commissioners as an ACP representative. At that time, he had little respect for the Joint Commission, but he developed into a strong supporter as a result of his experiences there. Ellis was neither the first nor the last commissioner to undergo this kind of conversion through experience.

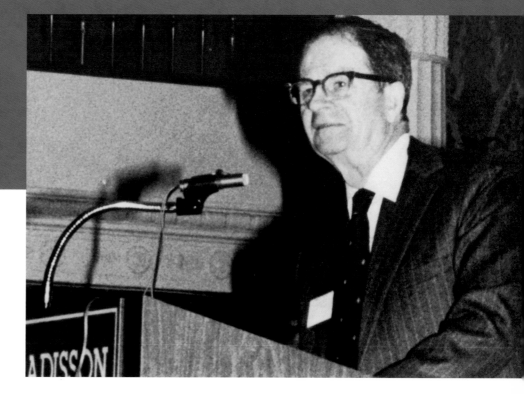

Westerman recalls how during this critical 1981 meeting Ellis used a technique that senior physicians liked to employ in medical staff meetings: They would remain silent while dissidents spoke and then they would ask questions. If the dissidents were shown to be careless, they would lose face. The tactic was essentially one of giving critics enough rope to hang themselves. At the outset, Ellis gave Sammons and McMahon the floor. They criticized Affeldt for being ineffective and a poor manager. Moser thought the attack was unfair and inappropriate, especially since Affeldt was not there to defend himself. He went immediately to Affeldt's defense and was distressed that he was alone at first. But then he was joined by Rollo Hanlon, George Dunlop (an ACS member from Worcester, Massachusetts, who was Ellis's traveling companion to Chicago), and several other commissioners, including McCallum.

Westerman, an AHA commissioner who served on the Planning and Organization Committee and who would soon chair it, marveled at Ellis's courtroom skill. Ellis criticized Sammons and McMahon for not having shared their knowledge of Affeldt's alleged management failures with them previously. He then proceeded to punch holes in their indictment. "You wouldn't treat a patient that sloppily," Ellis said, according to Westerman's recollection, "so why would you treat facts about Affeldt that way?" McMahon, a lawyer, had caucused with AHA com-

missioners prior to the meeting and knew that they were not all with him, so he grew silent, leaving Sammons to bear the brunt of the rebuttal.

Ellis and his allies saved Affeldt's job. The affair also showed a new assertiveness and independence on the part of the board, which was becoming more inclined to run the show and somewhat less inclined to be influenced by the corporate CEOs. Commissioners from the two colleges historically tended to be quite independent, chafing at perceived bloc-voting by their counterparts from the AMA and the AHA, who regularly caucused before board meetings to discuss the agenda — typically an excellent indication of how the meeting was likely to go. Of course, the CEOs dealt with opinions and political alignments within their constituencies that were often complex and dynamic, and their own job security could evaporate rapidly. The Joint Commission's by-laws gave CEOs floor privileges, but Ellis asked that they sit separately from the board at meetings. One commissioner recalls a meeting at which Jim Sammons offered some pieties and homilies, as was his tendency. Ellis looked at Sammons, who took great pride in being a tough, ornery Texan, and said, "Jim, where I come from in Arkansas, there's a saying about a statement like that — that's enough to make a buzzard puke." The remark broke up the room in laughter. Although differences in opinion were sometimes great, disagreements were rarely personal. Individuals sometimes locked horns at a meeting, then had a convivial drink together afterward.

As Ellis's two-year term as chairman drew to a close at the end of 1982, it was the AHA's turn to select a chairman from its ranks. Within the board's nominating committee, however, there was worry about Horace M. Cardwell, the AHA commissioner who was in line to succeed Ellis. Cardwell had sided with McMahon and Sammons in the failed coup. A few of his fellow AHA commissioners felt that Cardwell, who had been an administrator of a community hospital in Lufkin, Texas, since 1948, was entirely too close to the AMA. With McMahon pressing hard, however, Cardwell was approved as chairman in a very close vote, which sent a strong message. Moreover, two Affeldt supporters, Dunlop and McCallum, were elected vice chairman and treasurer, respectively. As the foregoing incidents suggest, politics in the health care field and at the Joint Commission can be rugged.

LITIGIOUS YEARS

In separate cases involving engineers and lawyers in the mid-1970s, the Supreme Court ruled that antitrust legislation applied to the professions. In 1976, the Federal Trade Commission initiated a preliminary investigation of the Joint Commission for suspected antitrust violations. The Joint Commission set standards related to hospital medical staffs' membership and privileges. In 1976, it was also named as a co-defendant in the *Wilk* case, a federal lawsuit that was brought by five chiropractors from different states against the AMA and other organizations. The chiropractors were seeking monetary damages, representation on the Joint Commission's board, and eligibility for medical staff membership. *Wilk* was the most enduring of a number of antitrust suits in which the Joint Commission was named a defendant, including ones filed by psychologists, podiatrists, nurse anesthetists, as well as individual doctors who had been denied staff privileges.

Eleanor Wagner, who had previously been an AHA staff attorney, came to the Joint Commission in 1976 as its first in-house counsel. She was hired with the expectation that she would be a generalist, but within a year most of her time was taken up by the various antitrust cases. She worked with Daniel Schuyler, who was the outside general counsel. While there were numerous defendants besides the Joint Commission and the AMA, the AMA's counsel was

lead counsel in defending the Wilk and other chiropractic antitrust suits. The AMA and other defendants were accused of having engaged in a conspiracy
to coerce or encourage doctors to boycott chiropractors. The AMA regarded chiropractic as quackery and
built its defense around its canon of ethics and the
protection of patients. The Joint Commission was
accused of being a willing tool in the AMA's alleged
conspiracy by limiting medical staff membership in
the hospital accreditation standards to physicians
and dentists.

In conjunction with the preliminary FTC investigation, the Joint Commission's lawyers developed a
defense theory that was based partly on the Medicare
law and partly on state institutional licensure laws.
Medicare conditions of participation for the most
part paralleled Joint Commission standards relative
to medical staffs. State laws, though they varied
somewhat, frequently tracked Joint Commission
standards on the subject of medical staffs. As long as
the Joint Commission was following both federal and
state laws, the counselors argued, it was not violating
antitrust laws.

In the early and mid-1980s, medical staff standards consumed a great deal of board time and generated a lot of internal controversy. They involved the
old question of where the power to credential staff
resided: with the executive committee of a hospital,
with the entire medical staff, or with specialized

departments. This dia-
logue grew tenser and
more tight-lipped with
the lawsuits pending.
Joint Commission staff
and board members had
to be careful with their
words because they did not know whether they might
be generating evidence for the plaintiffs.

In December 1982, six commissioners of the two
colleges and one from the ADA were outvoted by the
combined fourteen votes of AHA and AMA commissioners over the prospective use of the term "organized staff" in the *Accreditation Manual for Hospitals.*
"Why should physicians and others be outraged and
dismayed by the proposed revisions to the Medical
Staff Standards?" Rollo Hanlon asked his fellow surgeons in the ACS *Bulletin* of February 1983. He then
answered his question: "Primarily because they abol-
ish the word 'medical' wherever it appears, substitut-
ing for 'Medical Staff' the deliberately bland term
'Organized Staff.' And who is a member of the
Organized Staff? Why, anyone 'licensed for independent provision of patient care services.'"

The staff issue roiled organized medicine. "It was
far more than a turf issue," Robert Moser later wrote.
"It got to the root of the future role of the physician
as the advocate of the patient. This was a subtlety
that never seemed to penetrate some of the AMA and

AHA commissioners, or else they were beaten down into pragmatic acceptance by looming threats of litigation." There was much back-and-forth motion on the exact wording of the standards, though in December 1983, the board finally adopted a variation of what had been approved in late 1982, to go into effect the following July. They referred to a "single organized medical staff that has overall responsibility for the quality of the professional services provided by individuals with clinical privileges." Those privileges were defined as "permission to provide medical or other patient care services in the granting institution, within well-defined limits, based on the individual's professional license and his experience, competence, ability and judgment."

This meant that limited-licensed, non-medical "independent practitioners" could admit and care for patients in hospitals within the scope of their licenses, which were granted by states. As a practical matter, the modification did not erode medical authority in hospitals, as critics had feared. It provided greater flexibility and helped facilitate recognition of allied health professionals, whose training and contributions were increasingly valued by doctors.

Meanwhile, *Wilk* went through two trials, a jury trial and a bench trial, and numerous appeals over more than 10 years. In the end, the AMA was shown to have committed some antitrust violations, but the case against the Joint Commission was dismissed. By

the mid-1980s, the Joint Commission either won or settled on favorable grounds several other antitrust suits. It never was required to pay any monetary damages, though its legal defense was costly. Moreover, the Federal Trade Commission never took action against the Joint Commission.

That was not the end of the legal woes. Questions around the confidentiality of information that the Joint Commission received during surveys were also litigated in the 1980s. The pertinent laws were state, not federal, and they shielded certain kinds of peer review activities. For example, many states said that confidentiality applied in malpractice cases, since plaintiffs were able to obtain relevant facts in other ways, but said the shield did not apply in cases where doctors sued after they had been dismissed from staffs, since they had no other way to obtain relevant facts. (Aggrieved doctors brought hundreds of cases against hospitals in the early 1980s.)

For the Joint Commission, a key question was whether the peer review statutes applied to communications between it and accredited organizations. If these statutes did not apply, it would be difficult to have "candid communications" with institutions. In the *Niven* case, which involved medical malpractice, a subpoena was issued for Joint Commission documents pertaining to Northwestern Medical Center in Illinois. On the advice of counsel, Affeldt did not respond. As anticipated, the trial court issued Affeldt

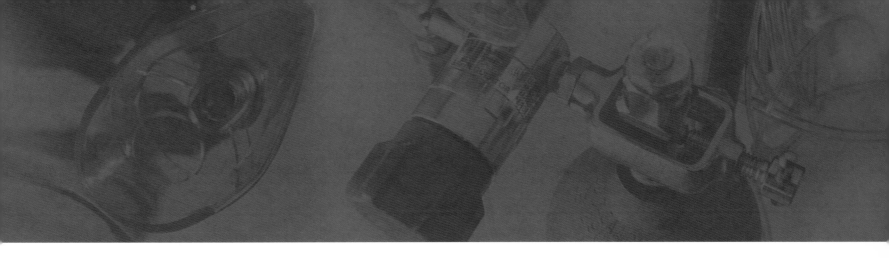

a contempt citation and, knowing that he planned to appeal, fined him nominally. In 1985, the Illinois Supreme Court ruled that the Illinois shield law did indeed apply, so Affeldt was cleared of contempt. *Niven* was a significant decision. Subsequent court rulings in Florida, New York and Texas essentially came to the same conclusion.

DEVELOPMENTS IN STANDARDS AND PROGRAMS

The previously discussed controversy over medical staffs was part of a larger process of revision of survey standards, which many constituents viewed as too regulatory. In a review of Affeldt's presidency in 1986, *Perspectives* described the process's guiding principles: "JCAH standards should relate as directly as possible to the quality of care and to the quality of the environment in which care is provided; they should represent consensus on the state of the art; they should, to the greatest extent possible, state objectives rather than mechanisms for meeting objectives; and they should be reasonable and surveyable." The new standards emphasized establishment of systematic quality assurance programs, improved management structures, and guidelines for competence-based practice. They also attempted to integrate the objectives of the various accreditation programs into a more unified system. For example, the language adopted to describe quality assurance was virtually the same for all accreditation programs.

In 1982, the two-year accreditation cycle was replaced by a three-year cycle for all programs except long-term care. The longer period between surveys obviously gave facilities more time to prepare, though it did not lower their costs on an annualized basis, as surveyor fees rose significantly at the same time. After awarding accreditation to a facility, the Accreditation Committee decided whether survey findings warranted contingencies, which were monitored through a variety of mechanisms, including written progress reports and focused follow-up evaluations by Joint Commission surveyors.

The Joint Commission likewise placed an even greater emphasis than before on its consultative and educational role. Hospitals enrolled their staffs in courses given by Joint Commission staff to help prepare them for survey. Moser saw a potential conflict of interest in being "advisor and consultant" as well as "regulator and accreditor," but the board felt that the two functions could be maintained as distinct entities. In fact, a large consulting industry had grown up around helping hospitals meet Joint Commission standards and prepare themselves for surveys. Former Joint Commission staff members and surveyors heavily populated this industry. Since there clearly was a market for such services and since sharing information and knowledge had always been central to the Joint Commission's mission, it made sense for it to offer consulting services, too.

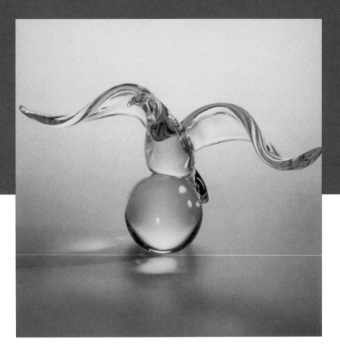

◀ **This beautiful Stuben eagle is a gift presented to outgoing chairs of the board of commissioners.**

Affeldt and other Joint Commission representatives also gave presentations at international symposia and found a great deal of interest in the Joint Commission's work. In 1983, the board restated its opposition to accrediting facilities outside the U.S. but endorsed responding to requests for education and consultation surveys that merely assisted facilities in determining their compliance with Joint Commission standards. Indeed, many countries were beginning to develop accreditation programs of their own and were using Joint Commission standards as models. Foreign delegations also periodically visited Joint Commission headquarters in Chicago or sought its advice. In the mid-1980s, the Joint Commission along with several other organizations and foundations sponsored large international symposia on quality assurance. In 1985, the board approved accepting a seat on the board of a new organization that had been registered in Sweden, the International Society for Quality Assurance (ISQA). A Joint Commission survey of King Fahad Hospital in Riyadh, Saudi Arabia, which treated many American

citizens as well as Saudis, led the board in 1986 to permit some exceptions to its former blanket prohibition on accrediting foreign hospitals. This modification aroused vocal opposition, in this instance, from Rollo Hanlon, though he failed to persuade his own ACS commissioners.

Another key aspect of the more rigid regime was the introduction in 1983 of a tailored survey process. Under it, there was a single comprehensive survey for health care organizations that offered more than one type of accredited health care service. All of an organization's services could be surveyed at the same time by a team of appropriately qualified surveyors.

Multihospital systems were proliferating in these years, as a result of the rapid growth of for-profit hospital chains and consolidations and acquisitions by not-for-profit hospitals. Consequently, the Joint Commission, with help from Kellogg Foundation grants, developed a survey process and modified standards to address the unique needs of multihospital systems.

In 1981, the Joint Commission received another Kellogg Foundation grant to develop standards and a self-assessment for hospice programs to care for terminally ill patients and their families. A grassroots hospice movement had been taking root in the United States, inspired by the hospice movement that began in England in the 1960s. Jim Roberts hired Barbara McCann, who had been the director of a government-funded hospice demonstration project, to direct the Joint Commission's hospice project. Over the next couple years, McCann conducted research, ran six invitational conferences, and staffed a task force to draft standards that were widely reviewed in the field.

Board members, particularly doctors, began to recognize that hospice should be legitimized through an accreditation program of its own. McCann recalls a difficult set of board meetings in 1983 in which there was a sharp difference of opinion between doctors and hospitals. Doctors were in favor of hospice accreditation because they felt the terminally ill were not being cared for properly. H. Robert Cathcart, an AHA commissioner who was the longtime CEO of the distinguished Pennsylvania Hospital in Philadelphia, did not believe that hospitals needed another set of standards. Don Avant recalls that Cathcart was on the task force that created the hospice standards and then he was the only one to vote against establishment of the new program. Cathcart was concerned that hospice standards would lead to further departmentalization in hospitals. Cathcart was a "lumper, not a splitter," observes Avant, who also notes that hospitals were generally leery of adding programs.

The new program that was approved by the board in August 1983 and began to operate in 1984 was designed for independent hospices and for hospice programs based in hospitals, home health agencies,

long-term care and psychiatric facilities. To be eligible for survey, a hospice program was required to offer interdisciplinary team services in both home care and inpatient settings. The teams normally included nursing, physician, psychological/social work, spiritual, volunteer, and bereavement services. Hospice standards and surveys had a number of innovations, including spiritual services, interviewing patients themselves, and examining continuity of care across settings. The standards that were adopted represented a consensus among various providers and a significant contribution on the part of the Joint Commission to the legitimization and fostering of hospice care in the United States.

O'LEARY APPOINTMENT

In March 1984, John Affeldt informed the board that he would retire by August 1986. Affeldt was comfortable with what he had accomplished in the demanding role of president; he also wanted to take life a little easier. (Like his two predecessors, Affeldt did not completely retire, for he continued to work part-time as consultant after leaving the Joint Commission.) The board had plenty of time to think about the Joint Commission's needs and to conduct a broad search for the next president. In August, an executive search firm was hired and a search committee was named. It was chaired by Ceylon "Burr" Lewis, a commissioner from the ACP, and included four other

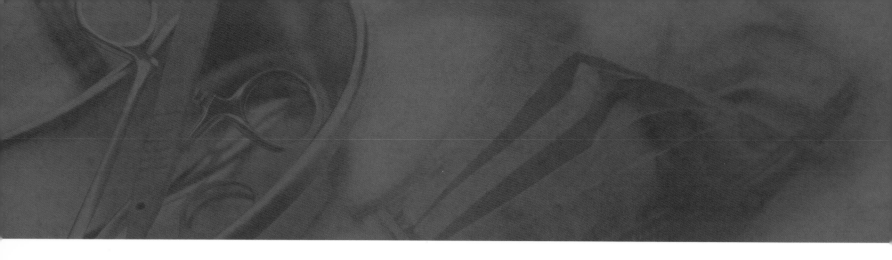

commissioners and the CEOs of the five corporate members, including John M. Coady of the ADA. Karen Timmons, named vice president of administration in 1985, staffed the committee.

The Joint Commission presidency is one of the most prominent in the health care field. When the job description was written in 1984, the Joint Commission's annual operating budget was $22 million. It had 411 employees, 243 in Chicago and another 168 surveyors in the field. Its occupant was asked to attend and frequently to speak at a variety of professional meetings, and such engagements consumed about a quarter of the president's time. "Personal and professional relationships with key contacts in the industry provide invaluable assistance," noted the job description. The president also had to stay abreast of the changing health care environment, especially state and federal regulations as well as the needs of customers and consumers. "The incumbent is challenged to guide and direct the JCAH membership and staff during a time of many changes in the industry. Vision is required to determine strategic options, diplomacy is required to secure support from the member organizations, and management expertise is required to implement those strategies selected."

Dennis O'Leary had come to public prominence in early 1981 by sheer circumstance. He was the spokesman for George Washington University

Hospital in the days following the attempted assassination of President Ronald Reagan and gave periodic televised briefings on the President's condition, answering questions from the media. He did all this candidly, calmly, and personably. O'Leary's demeanor had impressed many viewers, including as it happened, Alex McMahon's daughter, who one evening heard her father bemoan the fact that they had to find a new president for the Joint Commission. "How about that doctor who was on television when the president was shot?" she asked. Her father had also been impressed with O'Leary. Both the AHA and the AMA formally commended O'Leary for his effective communications during the crisis, and he had been invited to sit on advisory groups at the AHA and the AMA, where he had become acquainted with McMahon and Sammons.

The day after hearing his daughter's suggestion, McMahon called O'Leary to ask whether he would be interested in the Joint Commission presidency. He reached O'Leary at home because he was running a high fever from a kind of viral encephalitis. "In a moment of weakness," O'Leary later teased, he said that he would. A few months later, Jim Sammons approached him, too. By May, O'Leary had passed through the interview process and was offered the job.

O'Leary recalls that in his short interview with the search committee, he could not have been "more outrageous." He was happy at George Washington

Dennis O'Leary had come to public prominence in early 1981 by sheer circumstance... in the days following the attempted assassination of President Ronald Reagan.

and was not at all sure that he wanted the Joint Commission job, about which he knew little. So it was easy for O'Leary, who took pride in being a straight shooter, to be particularly blunt about the Joint Commission — he said it needed to be totally rebuilt. When the job offer came, it was clear that the search committee must have agreed with him.

O'Leary grew up in Kansas City, where his maternal grandfather, a physician, had helped found a major local hospital. O'Leary received his undergraduate degree from Harvard in 1960 and his medical degree from Cornell in 1964. He trained in internal medicine at the University of Minnesota Hospital and at Strong Memorial Hospital in Rochester, New York, and served at the Walter Reed Army Institute of Research in Washington. Board-certified in internal medicine and hematology, O'Leary was recruited to George Washington University Medical Center in 1971 as a specialist in blood clotting. Within six months of his arrival, he wrote a critique of the house-training program for his chairman, who promptly asked him to fix the problem. That marked his initiation in administration.

O'Leary chaired the medical staff executive committee for more than a decade, and he was dean for clinical affairs at the medical school from 1977 to 1986. He became a full professor of medicine in 1980, helping to organize and serving as vice president of the George Washington University Health Plan, an early academic HMO. In addition, he was president and chairman of the board of the District of Columbia Medical Society and a founding member of the National Capital Area Health Care Coalition.

When O'Leary formally accepted the presidency at the Joint Commission in August, he left behind a few patients in Washington. But he did not bother to obtain a medical license in Illinois, knowing he would not have time to practice. Instead, he lived vicariously off the practice of his wife, Margaret, who was an emergency medicine physician.

AGENDA FOR CHANGE
After his appointment, O'Leary was invited to a board retreat in September at Long Boat Key, Florida. Board retreats, which had been introduced by Affeldt, gave people a break from routine matters and allowed them to think longer term. It permitted informal discussions and fostered good will and friendship. People often brought their spouses and sometimes their children.

On the first morning of the retreat, John Affeldt and Jim Roberts put on the table the idea of a more performance-based accreditation process. Roberts talked about having clinical indicators as measurements of quality. O'Leary, who agreed with this direction, recalls that the board initially went "nuts" at the idea, dashing his high hopes. During a break in the meeting, however, Affeldt and Roberts reassured each other — and O'Leary — that the board was actually buying into the idea. Hearing these voices of experience, O'Leary realized that acceptance was all relative. Following the retreat, Affeldt, Roberts and O'Leary worked together to extract nuggets of truth about what needed to be done. Roberts, who had himself hoped to fill the presidential role, was encouraged to stay on as vice president for accreditation by board members and by O'Leary, who respected Roberts and shared his views. They were close collaborators on all that was to follow over the next several years.

At the December board meeting, the fruits of their combined labors were presented to the board as "Consensus Statements Emanating from 1985 BOC Retreat." There were 10 statements in all, but the first set the tone: "JCAH's attention to quality is its unique characteristic. While the historical focus of JCAH standards has been on a facility's organization and physical structure and its management of administrative and clinical functions, it is also essential that JCAH pursue means to link clinical markers to the survey process." Among the other statements were continuing to move toward flexible standards; assessing institutional competence, not the competence of individuals; increasing educational and consulting efforts; improving the credibility of the survey and the accreditation decision-making process; making the Joint Commission the principal repository of current knowledge on how to measure quality of care; and considering a substantial increase in survey fees. They also presented a set of assignments, or specific steps toward implementation.

The board "commended staff for the excellent synthesis of the deliberations of the retreat," the minutes recorded. Then the board voted to approve the consensus statements and assignments with minor changes. The process progressed further in April 1986, when Affeldt and O'Leary presented an issue paper to the board entitled, "An Agenda for Change." (According to plan, Affeldt retired after the meeting.) They had previously presented this paper to the Executive Committee, the Accreditation Committee, and the Standards-Survey Procedures Committee.

By the fall, to O'Leary's delight, the full board had signed off on the "Agenda for Change." This rubric was announced in a long article in the November/December issue of *Perspectives*. "The identification of specific clinical indicators will be under intense development during the next few years," the article explained. "This project is intended to refine or delete many organizational structure and function standards that now exist in Joint Commission standards manuals, with a stricter focus on standards that are demonstrably important to the provision of quality care." The development of an indicator system would begin with hospitals, because hospitals were in

6 | Joint Commission Sets
Accreditation | Agenda for Change

Clinical and organizational performance will be the focus of a new evaluation methodology now under development at the Joint Commission and scheduled to become part of the accreditation process in about five years.

The innovative system of performance evaluation, which centers on measures of health care quality as derived from clinical and organizational indicators, is the most far-reaching item on the "agenda for change" announced by Dennis S. O'Leary, MD, President of the Joint Commission. The agenda will involve the Joint Commission in a variety of related initiatives as well:

- Ongoing communication of clinical information and performance data from each health care organization surveyed to the Joint Commission corporate office, and feedback of comparative performance information to the organization.

- Revision of standards to address major current issues such as risk management and undercare.

- An expansion of Joint Commission educational initiatives.

The performance data will become part of an aggregate database which will make it increasingly possible, with time, to profile major delineations of quality of care using national and regional norms as reference points for comparison. The standards revision project has already resulted in the proposal of new standards explicitly addressing risk management and undercare. Based on field review comments, these proposed standards are undergoing further revision prior to further field review. The educational initiative has been discussed in detail in the July/August and September/October issues of *JCAH Perspectives*.

The patient-centered performance evaluation system will be the subject of an extensive developmental project that will be conducted at the Joint Commission over the next five years. This evaluation system is the centerpiece of the Agenda for Change and represents a completely new approach in analyzing health care quality and in assisting health care organizations to assure that quality care is being provided.

JCAH Perspectives November/December 1986

Background

Major changes in the financing of health care delivery and the creation of a competitive environment for providers have sparked demands for a new health care quality evaluation system, according to Dr O'Leary. The establishment of the prospective payment system has given rise to public concerns that altered payment incentives may adversely affect the quality of care, particularly in a resource-limited environment. This creates a need for scientifically sound and effective evaluation methodologies to monitor and identify incipient quality of care problems. The need for a new system has been identified in several quarters. "In the private sector, the purchasers of care are concerned not only about the cost but also the quality of care their employees receive," said Dr O'Leary. "Insurance companies, too, must weigh the quality of the care they pay for and in some cases provide. And when quality of care becomes a major public policy issue, the government responds to the public accountability imperative, which creates political and regulatory pressure for more exact measures of quality."

The development of the clinical indicator system is timely. The methodology for measuring clinical performance, at least in small systems, is now being described. And the computer technology necessary to apply the new methodologies to large systems, such as hospitals, is now available.

The New Evaluation System

Joint Commission staff who are developing the new evaluation system foresee the need for surveyed organizations to provide several kinds of data to the Joint Commission: This would include descriptive information about the type and volume of health care services provided as well as performance information based on a system of clinical and organization performance indicators.

The descriptive information will focus on types of services provided in a specific organization, on past and present patterns of problems associated with these services and on the volume of important services provided. The descriptive information

---

the best position to adapt to the new system and because hospital services involved the greatest risk and most complicated forms of care. However, the Joint Commission anticipated that it would soon thereafter develop a similar kind of outcomes system for nonhospital organizations.

The shift to measuring performance and clinical outcomes as the right way to measure quality was in effect a return to Codman's "End Result Idea," though the rehabilitation of Codman's role was to take a bit longer. A full explanation of why this shift occurred when it did could well be the subject of a separate chapter or even an entire book. But a brief — and necessarily superficial — explanation can be found in the confluence of certain ideas, technology and economics, which combined with gnawing doubt and frustration about existing standards and methodology.

In Codman's day, some of the key ideas about quality in health care originally derived from engineering. But many scientific advances occurred in medicine after World War II, and doctors naturally focused on these advances, not theory about assessment of health care quality. Meanwhile, W. Edwards Deming and Joseph M. Juran reconceputalized quality and its achievement in industry. During their long careers, they profoundly affected industrial production, first in Japan and then in America. Philip B.

Crosby, another influential quality expert from industry, also taught about the importance of systems knowledge and improvement, the drawbacks of inspections, and the need for statistical quality control. In the 1960s, Avedis Donabedian, a physician and student of public health, through his studies of nursing, gave weight to outcomes in addition to process and structure in assessing quality of care. He became an important bridge between old and new ways of thinking about health care quality. In the

QHR

Providing Quality Solutions for Healthcare

◄ *Quality Health Resources was established as a subsidiary of the Joint Commission to provide technical assistance to the health care field, particularly relating to the accreditation process.*

1970s and 1980s, interest in the theory of health care theory gradually began to revive — and with it an interest in what could be learned from other industries.

Empirical studies, which were made possible by advances in computer hardware and software, were allowing public health experts in academia and government to dissect and analyze large amounts of data. Among their findings was significant variation in treatment and outcome by geographical region, income, and race. These findings raised questions in turn about the consistency and quality of care and about under-utilization of the health care system by disadvantaged individuals. And with health care costs consuming a growing proportion of public and private spending, government and business were increasingly interested in measuring the effectiveness of health care spending. So, the public and private markets were also beginning to ask questions about how to measure quality.

A related change early in O'Leary's tenure was the creation of a subsidiary, Quality Health Resources, Inc., (QHR) as the home for technical assistance to the field, including pre-survey consultation services. Its board consisted of the executive officers of the board of commissioners. O'Leary felt that it was essential that the Joint Commission pro-

vide consulting services and that having a separate subsidiary would help deal with the perceived conflict of interest among some health care providers. Institutions were informed that they would not receive special treatment if they contracted with this service, and consultants for QHR were not permitted to obtain accreditation reports from the Joint Commission. If they wanted to see a confidential survey, they had to obtain it from the organization seeking accreditation.

And the need for consulting services was obvious. By 1986, the hospital program had 2,600 standards and the accreditation manual was 313 pages long. Although the Joint Commission's standards reflected the consensus of opinion among health care professionals, the specialization of the field had meant that the standards had become frustratingly detailed and excessively burdensome — threatening to topple under their own weight. Even some of those most intimately involved in the standard-setting process sometimes doubted their continued relevance, though the move toward more flexible standards in the early 1980s had eased these frustrations a little. Health care providers *wanted* the Joint Commission to shift the survey emphasis to results.

The redoing of standards was a highly ambitious goal, but O'Leary possessed a great deal of energy and imagination — and he had full confidence in his staff.

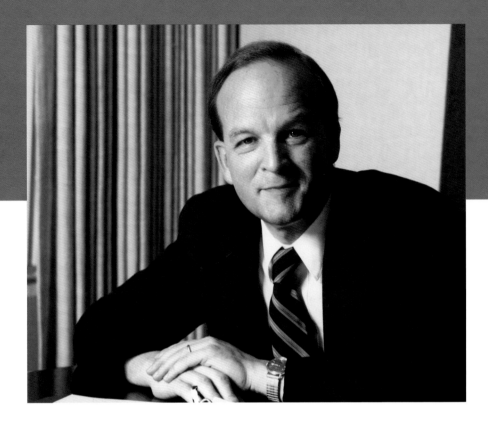

O'Leary had been impressed with the management team he inherited and retained most of it, adding a new vice presidential position that oversaw the divisions of education and publications and was filled by William F. Jessee. Trained in pediatrics and preventive health and with a strong academic and government background, Jessee was an early proponent of a systems approach to quality assurance and a friend of O'Leary. He had written extensively on educational methods for integrating quality assurance activities and clinical practice.

O'Leary refocused his management team on what he saw as its three major purposes: to develop policy, to share information so everyone on the team was apprised of key initiatives, and to answer questions and handle key issues. It was soon clear to the staff and the commissioners that O'Leary was interested in digging deep into Joint Commission operations — and that they would be pushed to the limits of their abilities to reach their goal.

▲ *Hired as an agent for change in 1986, Dennis O'Leary has overseen much change and growth during his 15 years as president.*

Changes and Challenges in a Dynamic Environment

CHAPTER FOUR

1986 - 2001

Staff members who were present in 1986 recall the Joint Commission as a small, sleepy organization compared to what it has become. Over the last 15 years, standards and programs have been added, eliminated and fundamentally revised; staff, budgets and public representation on the board have expanded; and external scrutiny and public accountability and disclosure have grown. All of this has taken place against the backdrop of a rapidly changing health care environment.

AN AGENT OF CHANGE

The board of commissioners hired Dennis O'Leary as an agent of change, though it is worth recalling that none of his predecessors — Edwin Crosby, Kenneth Babcock, John Porterfield, or John Affeldt — had been hired by earlier boards as caretakers. Naturally, the personalities, styles, and political and managerial skills of the administrative heads have varied, but all have been intelligent, hard working and dedicated. O'Leary's tenure, currently at 15 years, has been longer than that of any of his predecessors. But there have been times when his job security, too, has been shaky.

In a time of turmoil in the upper echelons of the health industry, O'Leary's longevity in office suggests considerable political skills. The CEOs of the member organizations have all turned over completely during his tenure, as have the board members. That turnover may have enhanced O'Leary's ability to set direction, pursue his central vision of focusing on outcomes, and provide continuity without inertia. Over the years, O'Leary has pushed and prodded the board, trying to move it to consensus, overcoming resistance with patience and persistence. O'Leary says that boredom has never been a problem for him as president. "There's one set of bullets whizzing by your head after another," he says, humorously confirming that the issues before the Joint Commission over the past 15 years have been diverse, important, and relentless.

During his "honeymoon," O'Leary moved on several fronts simultaneously. O'Leary had been a recent customer of accreditation at George Washington University Medical Center. He believed that the Joint Commission's staff did not adequately appreciate what it meant to be a service organization, and he sought concepts and assistance from the business world. He hired a consulting firm to provide training in customer service, and more rigorous financial management and planning, and he led the staff in an exercise to identify corporate values.

O'Leary also laid the foundation for revising standards, as called for in the Agenda for Change. At the end of 1986, the board appointed a steering committee to coordinate the Joint Commission's initiative to incorporate clinical and organizational indicators into a revised accreditation process, which was expected to take three to four years. The steering committee, whose chairman was Burr Lewis, was comprised of six board members plus outside experts Paul Griner from the University of Rochester, Stephen Shortell from Northwestern University, John Wennberg from Dartmouth Medical School, and Lincoln E. Moses from Stanford. Griner and Shortell were known for their research on the effects that variations in organizational structure had on clinical outcomes. Wennberg was known for his research on geographical variations in surgical practice, while Moses provided expertise on data systems. Paul Batalden joined the committee in 1990 as the fifth outside expert.

O'Leary, Jim Roberts, and James Prevost, who had formerly been director of standards development and who now became the first director of research and development, pursued foundation grants to support research into the development of organization performance measures known as indicators. The Robert Wood Johnson Foundation came through with the initial grant of $200,000. Over the next several years, this effort was also supported by grants from the American Cancer Society, Johnson & Johnson and the Kellogg, Hartford, and Prudential Foundations. But outside funding never completely covered the costs and the shortfall had to be met out of operating revenues. In 1987, task forces were established to formulate clinical indicators in two areas of hospital care, obstetrics and anesthesia. Both of these task forces were fruitful, producing results that were ready for testing in the field by 1990. Another task force, aimed at identifying hospital-wide clinical indicators, became bogged down and was disbanded in 1990.

Meanwhile, a fourth task force on organization and management indicators adopted principles of continuous quality improvement (CQI), which soon became fundamental to the revision of all standards. W. Edwards Deming, an American engineer, had taught CQI to the Japanese after World War II. The underlying concept was that quality was not an optimal level of performance that could be attained by

> CQI offered the promise of improving care, but also of saving money, an attractive objective at a time when annual increases in the cost of health care exceeded cost increases in the rest of the economy.

locating and removing "bad apples," but something to be continually improved through the study and refinement of processes. Quality improvement depended more on education than inspection, but it certainly relied on carefully measuring performance through statistical methods. CQI emphasized learning, collegiality, and organizational leadership, but it also required statistical measurements of performance to establish priorities for future improvements. CQI required that leaders invest time and money in the process and create an organizational culture that made quality a top priority.

After proving their theories in Japan, Deming and other American gurus of quality abroad were recog-nized as prophets in their own land, where, in the 1980s, American manufacturers themselves started to adopt the principles of CQI, sometimes known as total quality management (TQM). Experts on quality assurance in health care in the United States, including Paul Batalden, Stephen Schoenbaum, and Donald Berwick, saw that CQI had much to offer health care as well. CQI provided an escape from the inspectional/punitive box, changing the emphasis from individuals to systems and processes. It recognized that human beings inevitably make errors. By constantly working to improve processes rather than punish those who make errors, an organization could, it was hoped, reduce error rates and improve quality overall.

CQI offered the promise of improving care, but also of saving money, an attractive objective at a time when annual increases in the cost of health care exceeded cost increases in the rest of the economy. As it happened, several of the American enthusiasts for CQI either served on or advised the Joint Commission's task force on organization and management indicators, including Batalden, Berwick, and Shortell. They were the conduits through which CQI principles became intrinsic to the Agenda for Change.

Also in 1987, the board approved an increase in corporate members' contributions or dues from $15,000 per board seat to $20,000 per seat for the following year. They remained at $20,000 a seat until

1997, when they were quietly eliminated. By that time, they constituted a small fraction of total revenues. The largest source of revenue, of course, had long been survey fees, and the other revenue sources — publications, education, and consulting — were closely tied to the actual accreditation process.

In 1988, the Joint Commission implemented a new sliding-scale method of determining survey fees. It introduced a complex formula involving a combination of a base fee and variable charges that related to volume of inpatient days, outpatient visits and services. An underlying purpose of the new system was to produce greater equity, shifting more of the burden from smaller organizations to larger ones. More than half of accredited hospitals were small and rural. The AHA and its section on small and rural hospitals had reviewed and supported the new system before it was announced.

As soon as the new sliding scale went into effect, however, bigger hospitals experienced large increases, which they quickly protested. In defense of the new fee scale, O'Leary pointed out in *Perspectives* that the average hospital spent 20 times as much on marketing activities as it did on survey fees. Hospital managers felt that in a competitive environment they had no choice but to spend money on marketing activities. But they could try to do something about survey fees, and they had state associations and the AHA to assist them in this pursuit. Since the sliding-scale for-

mula was first instituted, it has been repeatedly tinkered with and modified.

In 1987, the Joint Commission changed its name from the Joint Commission on Accreditation of Hospitals to the Joint Commission on Accreditation of Healthcare Organizations. A name change had been considered before, going back to the establishment of the long-term care accreditation program in 1966, but the AHA had always opposed removing "hospitals" from the name. By 1987, the Joint Commission accredited 5,400 hospitals and more than 3,000 non-hospital organizations, and the AHA's argument crumbled, as hospitals continued to diversify into far more than acute care services.

A key factor in effecting a name change now, however, was that the Joint Commission was preparing to launch a new accreditation program in home care services. Many patients preferred to be at home, a less expensive alternative to hospitals and nursing homes, and they generally fared better there than in institutions. Moreover, Medicare had begun to pay for home care services and many medical technologies had become portable. Home care organizations resisted accreditation by hospital associations, and in 1987, the National League for Nursing created the Community Health Accreditation Program.

Retention of its old name would have placed the Joint Commission at a competitive disadvantage. In addition, the Joint Commission already had taken the first steps toward an accreditation program in managed care, another non-hospital field that was expected to grow in importance and where competition for external evaluation also existed.

After adopting the Joint Commission's new name in 1987, the board decided the following year to move to a new home, a decision that generated much greater internal controversy. The Joint Commission leased 75,500 square feet, comprising the 20th and 22nd floors of the John Hancock Building and parts of the ground and 34th floors, leasing additional space when the offices became overcrowded. Having staff located on non-adjacent floors was inconvenient and inefficient. The shortage of conference rooms for meetings and educational purposes meant that expensive off-site locations were rented with increasing frequency. Though a space planning study had been underway since 1986, the issue took on urgency in early 1988 when the Joint Commission was given a deadline to exercise its option on the 23rd floor.

As vice president for operations, Karen Timmons managed the planning effort as well as the subsequent move, though O'Leary took a great interest in both matters. They engaged a real estate broker, a space planning firm, and tax counsel to explore relocation of the Joint Commission offices and discussed ways to relieve problems of transportation and transition.

They soon decided that the best course was to leave Chicago for new headquarters that would be built-to-suit by a developer in Oakbrook Terrace, 25 miles west of downtown Chicago. The Joint Commission would own the property and building and would also have an option on an adjacent piece of land, on which it could expand in the future.

The thought of leaving downtown Chicago disturbed some commissioners, however, including Rufus K. Broadaway, who happened to be vice chairman at the time. An AMA representative, Broadaway accepted the necessity of moving out of the John Hancock Building, home since 1973, but he was appalled that a health care organization of national prominence such as the Joint Commission would decide to move to the "boonies." At the time, he recalls, there were still cows grazing in Oakbrook. Visiting commissioners had long taken pleasure in Chicago, a beautiful, cosmopolitan city, had their favorite hotels and restaurants, and often combined meetings at the Joint Commission with other business downtown.

Four out of the five corporate members (all but ACP) had headquarters in Chicago. The two colleges and ADA supported the prospective move to the suburbs. But at the AMA and the AHA, there was a feeling, not completely unfounded, that O'Leary wished to leave the city so that he would be under less immediate control and scrutiny by the corporate parents.

Timmons compares the move to Oakbrook to teenagers who grow up and want to get out of their

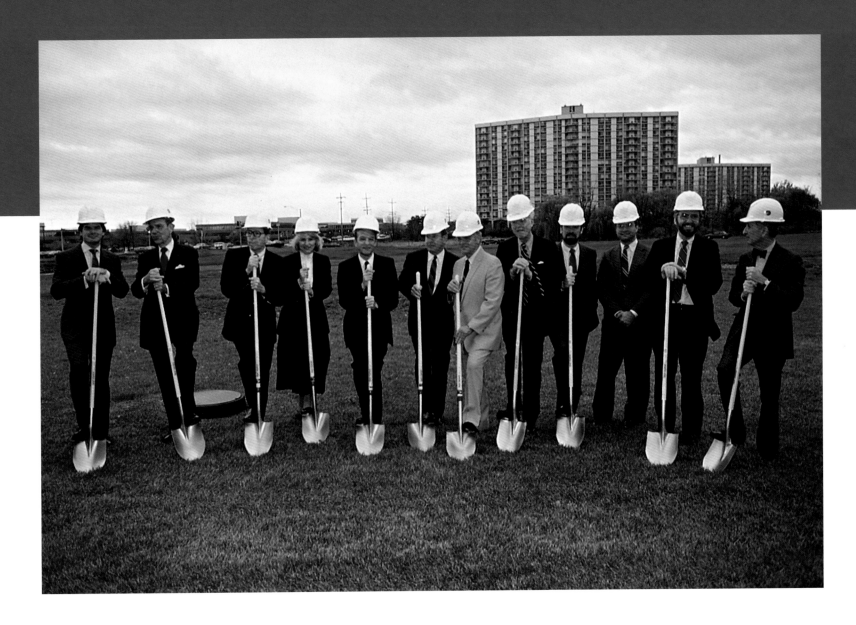

parents' house. O'Leary does not seem to regret that the CEOs of the corporate parents have been much less inclined to come to meetings at Oakbrook than they had been downtown. However, the primary reason for the move was clearly financial.

Commissioners felt obliged to get the most out of available revenues, three-quarters of which came from survey fees. For that reason, the AHA came around, but feelings ran high. At one meeting,

▲ *Dennis O'Leary, Karen Timmons, and members of the board of commissioners broke ground for new headquarters in Oakbrook Terrace in 1988.*

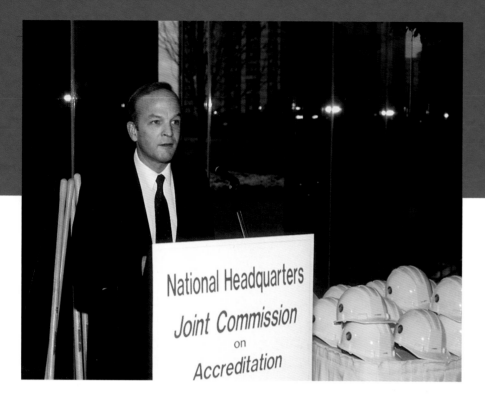

Broadaway and Burr Lewis nearly came to blows. Broadaway led a solid bloc of six AMA commissioners in voting against the move. (Another AMA commissioner was absent on the day of the deciding vote in July.) But the board approved the move.

Timmons oversaw the financing for the new offices through bonds issued by the city of Elmhurst, a neighboring city that, unlike Oakbrook Terrace, had the ability to issue bonds. Accrediting agencies were unfamiliar to bond insurers. So in lieu of bond insurance, the Joint Commission secured a letter of credit from the Commonwealth Bank of Australia, for which it paid a fee, as it would have for bond insurance. On October 12, 1988, the day the bonds were to close, a long article by investigative reporter Walt Bogdanich appeared on the front page of the *Wall Street Journal*. The article alleged that the Joint Commission was a poor regulator in that it failed to discipline slipshod hospitals. Bogdanich began with the tragic story of a patient who had died at an

accredited, but woefully inadequate hospital in New York City that subsequently closed. Bogdanich referred to the Joint Commission as "one of the most powerful and secretive groups in all of health care." He alleged that the Health Care Financing Administration (HCFA) failed to properly oversee the Joint Commission. (HCFA had been created to oversee Medicare, Medicaid and related medical quality care programs as part of a government reorganization when the Department of Health and Human Services was established in 1977.)

Bogdanich expanded his article into a book, *The Great White Lie*, published in 1991, a more general indictment of hospitals and medical care. Bogdanich was a harbinger of closer and more intense scrutiny by the press of failures, errors, and shortcomings in health care, particularly as they relate to patient safety. Such reporting, sometimes sensationalistic and soon including television, became a staple of contemporary journalism. Those who are depicted as villains, including the Joint Commission, doctors, and government and hospital officials, naturally find themselves vulnerable and easily become defensive.

The particular timing of Bogdanich's initial *Wall Street Journal* article could not have been worse for the Joint Commission. October 12, 1988, found Timmons and Harold Bressler, the Joint Commission's general counsel since 1985, meeting with a large group of bond lawyers, who asked whether the

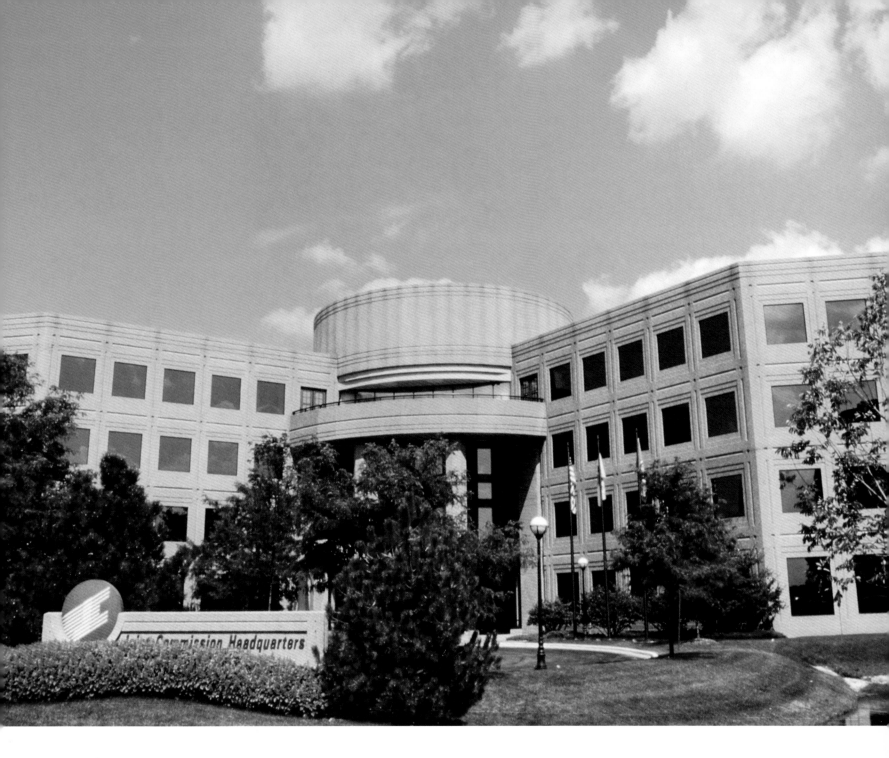

▲ *The Joint Commission's modern new headquarters has architectural references to Thomas Jefferson's Monticello.*

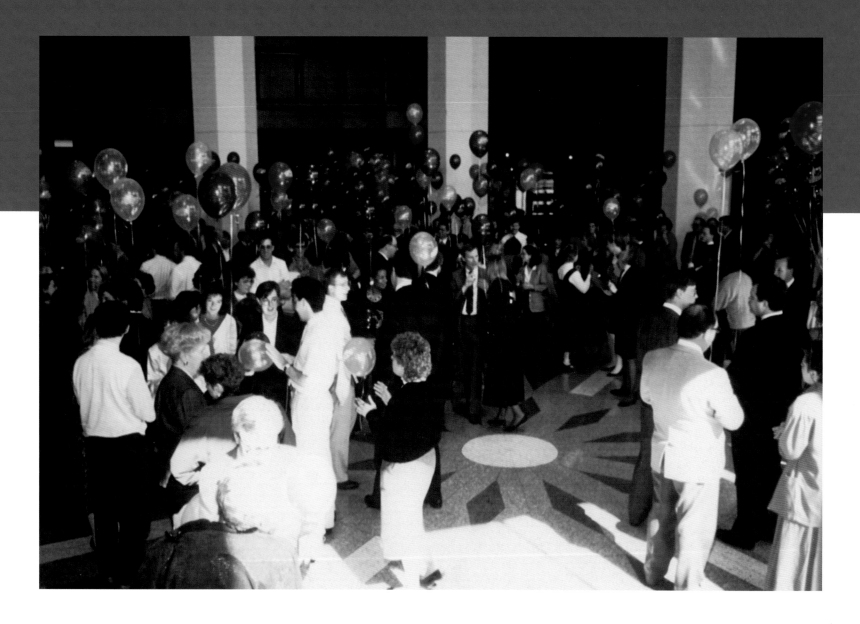

▲ *Staff and board members celebrate in the rotunda of the new headquarters at the official opening celebration on April 10, 1990. Though some had originally objected to the move, everyone was pleased and impressed with the new headquarters building.*

Joint Commission was even going to be in business in a year. The bank considered withdrawing its letter of credit. Efforts to reassure the bankers, including calls by O'Leary to Australia, awakening them in their beds, worked. The bank stood by the letter of credit, and the bonds were sold.

O'Leary took a personal interest in the design of the new headquarters, a modern, four-story 150,000-square-foot building with architectural references to

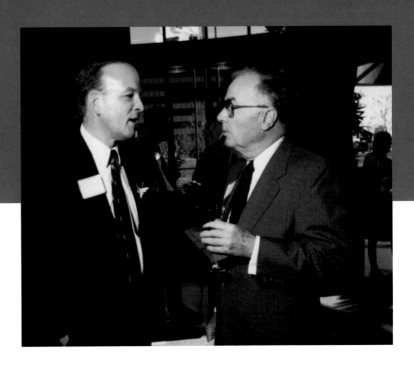

Thomas Jefferson's Monticello. The building includes a large boardroom, a conference center, and a four-level parking deck for employees and visitors. During construction, some employees were temporarily located in a nearby building while others remained downtown. The Joint Commission retained most employees through transportation subsidies, vanpools, and paying for moving expenses, but a small number decided not to relocate. Staff members appreciated the new building's efficient layout, which aided internal communications and cohesiveness. Coincidentally, when the building opened on April 10, 1990, Broadaway was board chairman. He graciously presided over the ribbon-cutting ceremony. By then, he recalls with good humor, all agreed the new building was beautiful.

HOME CARE, MANAGED CARE, AND MISSION

In O'Leary's early years, two new nonhospital programs were launched, home care and managed care, though they had very different fates. In late 1987, the board authorized initiation of home care accreditation surveys, using a comprehensive set of new standards that had been developed to address the entire spectrum of home care services, from traditional home health agencies to companies offering durable medical equipment services to those providing medicinal and nutritional home infusion therapy. It included for-profits and not-for-profits. The program, launched in June 1988, had been developed by Barbara McCann, who had previously founded the hospice program. McCann oversaw the recruitment and training of surveyors, all of whom were part-time and worked in the home care field.

Don Avant credits McCann with bringing the durable medical equipment providers into the fold. They were entrepreneurs whose interest in accreditation was primarily that it might give them a marketing edge, according to Avant. Their inclusion was controversial. State associations in home care, which were comprised of not-for-profits such as visiting nurses agencies, generally would not even let proprietary companies become members. McCann, in turn, credits Scotty McCallum, who was chairman at the time, for understanding the necessity of covering the full spectrum of home care for the benefit of patients. When an accreditation manual was published the following February, it included core standards and separate standards unique to each piece of the industry. This pioneered an approach to standards that other Joint Commission programs later adopted.

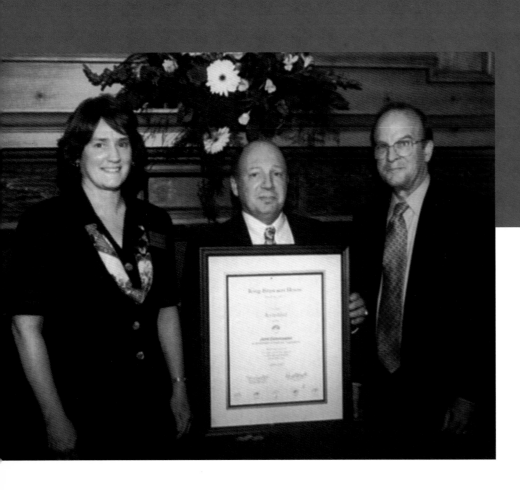

revenues of $22,600,000 while the hospital program had a total volume of 2,358 surveys and revenues of $39,100,000.

From the outset, O'Leary wanted the Joint Commission to evaluate managed care. Having been involved in the creation and operation of an HMO at George Washington, he believed that managed care was likely to grow. In the mid-1980s, states had begun to contract with managed care providers to run their Medicaid programs and were looking for third-party evaluations of their performance. The Joint Commission won a contract with the State of Ohio and subsequent contracts in several other states. From the beginning, however, the AMA expressed its reservations about accrediting managed care. Some AMA members and one AMA commissioner, Raymond Scalettar, were ready to live with managed care, but theirs was a minority view. Traditional fee-for-service doctors as a whole disapproved of managed care on ethical grounds, but also viewed it as an economic and political threat. And they did not want the Joint Commission to lend legitimacy to managed care through accreditation.

Nevertheless, in 1989 the Joint Commission quietly initiated a managed care accreditation program. It created an excellent set of standards drawn up by an advisory committee that included medical directors from several of the country's most highly regarded HMOs, including Kaiser-Permanente and Harvard

McCann knew that obtaining deemed status would increase the value of accreditation to customers, but deemed status was not granted by HCFA until 1993. Nevertheless, the Joint Commission's home care program was quick-off-the-mark, flexible, competitively priced, and broadly based. It soon developed into the largest accrediting agency in home care. By 1993, it had accredited more than 3,000 home care organizations, and by 1995, it was conducting more surveys on an annual basis than the hospital accreditation program. In revenues, the hospital program is substantially larger than home care because hospital surveys are more complex, take longer, and use physician surveyors primarily. The home care program, on the other hand, uses nurses and pharmacists primarily. In 1997, for instance, home care had a total volume of 3,373 surveys and

Community Health Plan. The program's launch was so quiet that *Perspectives* did not mention it. Just a year later, however, *Perspectives* did include a short report when the board voted to terminate the program. The article in the May/June 1990 issue explained that the "managed care field appeared reluctant to accept accountability for the full range of quality of care responsibilities." The article noted that most group and staff-model HMOs remained eligible for accreditation under the Joint Commission's ambulatory care standards. The article reported that the board had also voted to discontinue its hospice program, whose standards would be incorporated into other programs.

Explanations differ on how and why the two programs were ended. The terminations happened at a time when the board as a whole was concerned that the organization was over-extended financially and managerially. It was also a time when hospitals were getting anxious about worsening financial conditions, looming clinical indicators, a more regulatory environment, and increasing public disclosure. In 1986, HCFA had begun to publish individual hospitals' Medicare mortality data. The Joint Commission, which was committed to developing new performance indices, would undoubtedly face pressure to release its own data to the public.

O'Leary's "honeymoon" was certainly over by 1990 as operational issues moved to the fore. In the late 1980s, a significant backlog in survey reports had developed. Accreditation decisions and appeals had slowed down to a trickle, and there were many concerns from the field about the contents and effectiveness of standards and about the quality and consistency of surveyors. In 1988, the Joint Commission began to conduct opinion surveys of hospital CEOs to establish a baseline for its customers' level of satisfaction. It found that 38 percent of respondents felt that the Joint Commission had improved its performance over the previous five years, but 26 percent felt its performance had worsened, and another 26 percent perceived no change.

During the same meeting in which the managed care program was terminated, the board also considered discontinuing the long-term care program. Mary Tellis-Nayak, who was the program's director at the time, recalls being told by a vice president that the board was probably going to kill it. When the meeting ended, however, she was relieved to learn it had been spared. Tellis-Nayak notes that she ran the program on a shoestring. For example, she was a paid speaker at various conventions on quality improvement and quality assurance, so she was able to market the program while the Joint Commission paid for only a fraction of her travel expenses. The long-term care program at least managed to cover its costs.

Nursing homes were generally small, for-profit operations, though there were a few large not-for-profit and for-profit operations. Most nursing homes were in smaller regional chains or were "mom-and-pop"

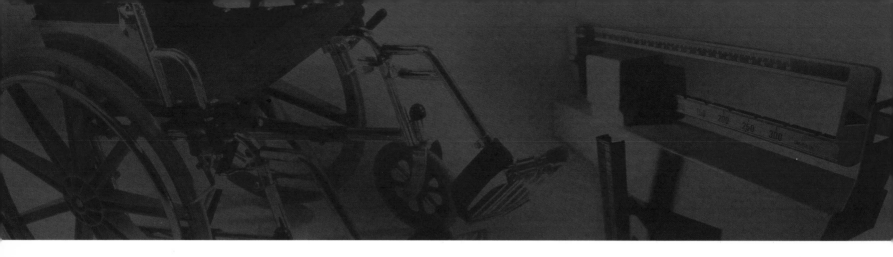

operations. Nursing homes were regulated by HCFA. The Joint Commission has never succeeded in obtaining deemed status for its long-term care program. Accreditation, which was strongly educational in orientation, has always appealed to the better facilities. Only a small proportion of all nursing homes has ever been accredited by the Joint Commission, and as recent government studies have shown, the quality of care in the nation's 17,000 nursing homes leaves a tremendous amount to be desired. According to a 1999 report by the U.S. General Accounting Office (GAO), more than one-fourth of nursing homes had deficiencies that "caused actual harm to residents or placed them at risk of death or serious injury." In the summer of 2000, an exhaustive study by the Office of Health and Human Services (HHS) reported that nursing homes were seriously understaffed. It recommended new federal standards and said that 54 percent of nursing homes currently fall below its proposed "minimum standard." These findings suggest that federal regulation of health care facilities is hardly a panacea.

Unlike the long-term care program, the hospice and managed care programs were not covering their costs. There were many hospice programs, but they were relatively poor and had difficulty affording accreditation. On the other hand, there were relatively few managed care organizations. They could afford accreditation, but lacked interest. The Joint Com-

mission had made a considerable investment in developing its standards for managed care, but HMOs were not lining up to be accredited. If their competitors in fee-for-service medicine did not have a rigorous quality review program, why should they?

The Joint Commission did sign up one major managed care organization just two months before the board pulled the plug. Daniel Dragalin, medical director of PruCare and a member of the Joint Commission's task force, had seen accreditation as an opportunity to differentiate his company in the marketplace. O'Leary still had hopes for the program and would have liked to stay the course, but reading the tea leaves from a board retreat in March, he recommended termination of the managed care program in May 1990.

It is important to note that the National Committee for Quality Assurance (NCQA) was also struggling to establish itself as an evaluator of managed care in these years. NCQA had been formed in 1979 by the leading managed-care trade associations to fend off federal regulation. By the late 1980s, a few of their leaders had come to the conclusion that NCQA had to become an independent body if it was ever to be seen as credible. James Doherty, the veteran CEO of the Group Health Association of America, later explained: "I argued that we must assume that wherever health care is provided on a prepaid basis and providers are placed at some financial risk, there is an inherent, natural, logical incentive to undertreat patients. To counter the endless charges of undertreatment leveled by organized medicine, HMOs needed to subject their operations to external review by an independent quality assurance body."

Consequently, in 1990, with assistance from a Robert Wood Johnson Foundation grant, NCQA reconstituted itself and became independent. HMOs were still represented on its board, but so were consumers and purchasers, that is, large employers. NCQA moved into the breach created by the Joint Commission's withdrawal and became a major player in quality assessment and accreditation in managed care and in public policy discussions as well. O'Leary acknowledges that NCQA would have been a formidable competitor even if the Joint Commission had remained in the field, though he believes that the decision to leave the managed care field was the worst strategic error during his tenure. In 1994, the board recognized its error when it launched an accreditation program for health care networks, where it competes with NCQA.

Consumer advocates sometimes challenged the Joint Commission's credibility on the grounds that it was dominated by health care providers. Following the publication of Bogdanich's article, Congressman Fortney H. "Pete" Stark of California, chairman of the House Ways and Means Subcommittee on Health, asked GAO to report on the adequacy of HCFA's

oversight of the Joint Commission. In June 1990, GAO reported on a number of problems and deficiencies. It recommended closer monitoring but also better coordination between HCFA and the Joint Commission. In response to sharp congressional criticism that it received during 1988 hearings on legislation concerning clinical laboratories, HCFA increased its annual volume of validation surveys of accredited hospitals from 50 to 250, a five-fold increase. As before, these surveys were contracted out to state health agencies. Moreover, HCFA's Medicare "conditions of participation" did not exactly correspond with Joint Commission standards. Validation surveys had never been a very effective way to monitor the Joint Commission.

The commissioners appreciated the contributions that public members had made to discussions of policy matters at the board level and on various task forces, and it was undoubtedly also true that public representatives enhanced the Joint Commission's legitimacy and credibility. Bill Beers encouraged an increase in the number of public members, as did O'Leary and the commission's chairman and vice-chairman, McCallum and Broadaway. However, the corporate members had no desire to sacrifice control in exchange for credibility. In late 1988 the board voted to add two more public members, raising board membership to 24. By limiting the public members' voting to issues other than by-laws, the control of the

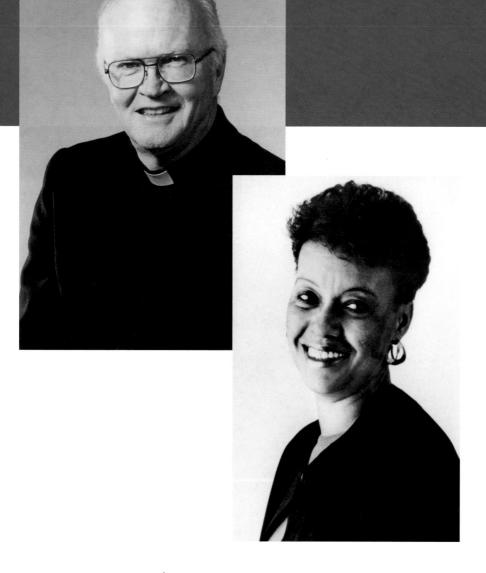

▲ *In 1989, Father William J. Byron, president of the Catholic University of America, and Carolyn O. Lewis, an executive with the Securities and Exchange Commission, were appointed to the Joint Commission's board as public members.*

corporate members was assured. (Corporate members cast their votes as blocs on by-laws: one identified AHA member casts seven votes, and one identified AMA member casts seven votes. By-law changes require three-fourths of the 21 votes of members, that is, *corporate* members, so either organization can block any by-law amendment or dissolution of the corporation, if that were to be proposed.)

Father William J. Byron and Carolyn O. Lewis were appointed commissioners in August 1989 and began to attend board meetings the following January. Byron, a Jesuit priest, had earned a doctorate in economics and was president of the Catholic University of America in Washington, D.C. He had served on a hospital board in Washington and was very experienced in accreditation in higher education. It also so happened that he had grown up in a medical family.

At the time of her appointment, Lewis was an executive with the Securities and Exchange Commission. Earlier in her career, she had served on a federal board that reviewed reimbursement disputes between health care providers and the government. Since 1975, she had also been a board member of a health care and community development organization in Washington. Lewis was the first African-American to become a commissioner.

Byron and Lewis were unintimidated by the technical questions that routinely came before

> **Having three public members reduced their isolation and made them easier to be heard, though there was still a way to go before the number of public members reached critical mass.**

the board. At times they were frustrated by the parochialism and self-interest that sometimes were in evidence, though they were impressed with the dedication, intelligence, and commitment to high ideals they saw as well. They understood their responsibility to raise questions and offer an outside perspective, to consider the organization's long-term condition, and to represent the public broadly. Having three public members reduced their isolation and made them easier to be heard, though there was still a way to go before the number of public members reached critical mass.

In 1990, Byron succeeded Beers as the public member on the Executive Committee, and in 1991, John K. Castle, succeeded Beers, on the board. Castle was a successful New York investment banker who had recently completed service as chairman of the board of New York Medical College. He was also a director of the United Hospital Fund of New York and had served as director of several hospitals. In 1991, Helen L. Smits succeeded Broadaway as chairman of the board, and as such became the first woman to serve in that capacity. Smits had joined the board as an ACP representative in 1989. She brought to the chairmanship a wealth of experience in hospital management, clinical medicine and health services research. Smits had taught medicine and epidemiology and public health at Yale; had been director of health standards and quality at HCFA; and was director at the University of

Connecticut Health Center when she assumed the Joint Commission chairmanship.

By 1990, there was considerable internal discussion about exactly whom the Joint Commission served. When he was asked that question in a forum, O'Leary reported in *Perspectives* early in 1990, he responded without hesitation, "the public." He did not mean that the Joint Commission had become a consumer advocacy group, though it talked to such groups. O'Leary recalled with pride the Joint Commission's origins in the hospital standardization program of the American College of Surgeons, which was created out of concern about "the quality of care in the nation's hospitals." But these were very different times. "The cost of care and resource constraints have created anxieties and frustrations for hospitals and

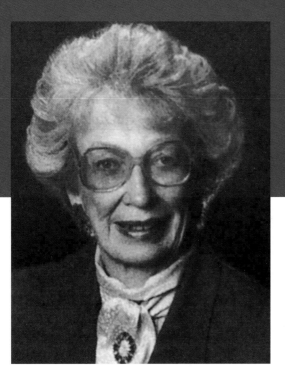

patients alike." Meanwhile, consumer groups and government were insisting on greater accountability by health care providers and accrediting bodies. Because accreditation stakes were much higher and because the Joint Commission was, through deemed status, carrying out a public responsibility, even becoming an arm of government in the view of many, hospitals regarded the Joint Commission more warily.

In 1990, the board continued to discuss whom the Joint Commission served and who its primary customers were. At a board retreat early in the year it was agreed "that the Joint Commission exerts its primary influence through the accreditation process and that it should therefore be fundamentally oriented to hospitals and other health care organizations." The board suggested that the mission statement, which had been revised two years before, be revised again, that it identify "*why* the Joint Commission exists, that it more explicitly identify the Joint Commission's primary customer (health care organizations), and that it emphasize the Joint

Commission's leadership role in developing and teaching quality improvement methods."

When a revised mission statement was approved in September, however, the public purpose was back on top and there was no mention of customers: "The mission of the Joint Commission on Accreditation of Healthcare Organizations is to improve the quality of health care provided to the public. The Joint Commission develops standards of quality in collaboration with health professionals and others and stimulates health care organizations to meet or exceed the standards through accreditation and the teaching of quality improvement concepts." Two years later, in 1992, the board removed the second sentence describing *how* the Joint Commission accomplished its mission because it felt that it detracted from its foremost purpose.

FURTHER BOARD EXPANSION, REVISED STANDARDS, AND RESPONSE IN THE FIELD

In 1992, with encouragement from individual board members and from O'Leary, the board agreed to expand further, adding three more public representatives and an at-large representative of the nursing profession. This brought the total to 28 seats. At the time this expansion took place, there was a proposal to reduce the size of the board by six seats — two each from the AHA and the AMA and one each from ACS and ACP. The two colleges were willing to surrender

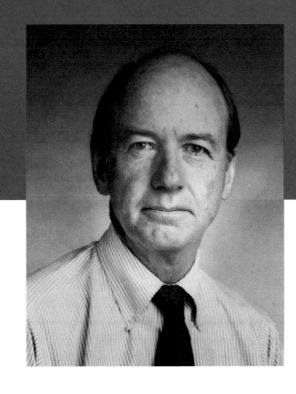

seats, provided the AMA and the AHA each gave up two of theirs, but the two associations declined. A separate proposal to delete the names of the corporate members from the Joint Commission letterhead also died — they are still listed there today. The board decided that the at-large nursing seat and one public member seat would be filled in 1993 and that the two remaining public seats would be filled in 1994.

Organized nursing had periodically sought representation on the board. These efforts had resumed in the early 1990s with a request for corporate membership from the American Nurses' Association. Since 1980, the AHA included a nurse among its representatives, first Barbara Donaho and subsequently Helen Ripple and Karen Ehrat. Now the board decided to add a nurse as an at-large member, not as a representative of any one nursing organization. The board's nominating committee conducted a search, as it did for public members, and selected Sally Ann Sample. Sample had been a member of ANA since completing her training in the late 1950s and had served on its board of directors from 1985 to 1987, but she was also a member of the American Organization of Nurse Executives and the National League for Nursing. She had served as ANA's representative on the hospital program's PTAC since 1987 and been its chair, and was therefore familiar with the Joint Commission. She had gotten to know John Helfrick of ADA during her service on the PTAC and Helfrick

had helped her understand the Joint Commission's political process. That understanding, which she communicated to nursing organizations, in fact, had been instrumental in helping to obtain the at-large seat for nursing in 1993.

As the at-large representative of the nursing profession, Sample, like the sole ADA representative on the board (John Helfrick from 1992 until 1999, and David Whiston since 2000), was drafted to serve on many standing committees and key task forces. She used her strong network of contacts in nursing to reach out for advice and assistance on a range of issues. Because of her close contact with the nursing profession, for example, she played an important role in alerting the board to the importance of addressing the use of patient restraints.

Dean O. Morton joined the board as a public member with Sample in 1993. Morton was executive vice president and chief operating officer of Hewlett-Packard Company and had been vice chair of the board of Stanford University Medical Center. In 1994,

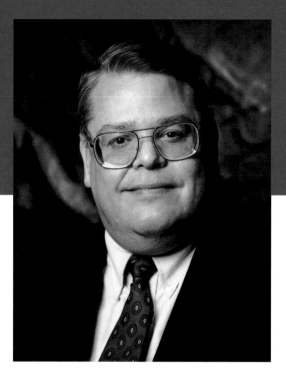

according to plan, two other public representatives joined the board, Alexander M. Capron and Charles H. McTier. A law professor at the University of Southern California, Capron is a leading expert in medical ethics and health policy. McTier is president of four philanthropic foundations in Atlanta, including the Robert W. Woodruff Foundation, all of which are interested in health issues.

While not the fundamental reconstitution of the board that consumer advocates and experts on corporate governance of not-for-profits might have preferred, the expansion of public representation on the board has had an effect. A former staff member notes that the public members have come to exercise influence far in excess of their numbers, simply because none of the representatives of corporate members want to appear to be opposing the public interest. Nevertheless, there were still some very rocky times ahead.

Meanwhile, the Agenda for Change was moving from research and theory to implementation and

practice. A partial revision of the hospital standards and manual was completed in 1992 and then a more extensive revision two years later. By the end of 1995, all other standards and manuals were revised as well.

The new standards were organized around function rather than structure; they included measurement of an organization's *performance* in providing care, not an organization's *capacity* to provide care; they required organizations to adopt continuous quality improvement principles, though the precise term was not used. Under Vice President Paul Schyve's supervision, most of the old standards were completely rewritten and a substantial number were eliminated, which meant that manuals were considerably shorter. The *1995 Accreditation Manual for Hospitals* included six new functional areas: patient rights and organizational ethics; care of patients; continuum of care; management of the environment of care; management of human resources; and surveillance, prevention and control of infection. All of these subjects had been covered in some fashion before, though not in a functional way.

In 1992, a new standard was added requiring that all hospitals have a policy prohibiting smoking. This generated a great deal of controversy and comment, though most of it occurred behind-the-scenes because by that time no doctor or hospital official wished to be seen as favoring smoking. O'Leary received more mail and phone calls on this new standard than he had on any other. Interestingly, the smoking prohibition in hospitals followed by six years a smoking ban the board had imposed on itself. That original prohibition had been championed by Sister Irene Kraus, a Catholic nun and hospital administrator who joined the board in 1982 as an AHA representative. Alan Nelson recalls that Sister Irene had been appalled to discover that an AMA commissioner puffed cigars at Joint Commission meetings. Sister Irene, Nelson notes, had not been reticent about expressing her feelings on this subject.

The survey process became more system-wide and cross-departmental, as well as more closely tailored to the individual organization. It involved more disclosure to the public of organization-specific results, including the number and nature of confirmed substantive complaints against accredited facilities, and the existence of Type 1 recommendations. (Such recommendations follow discovery of a serious shortcoming in a specific performance area; the recommendations must be met within a stipulated time frame in order for an organization to maintain its accreditation.) Organizations supplied more documentation in advance of visits, giving surveyors more time to interact with staff.

The new survey process placed greater emphasis on education and consultation, and provided for on-site identification of survey findings and exit interviews with top management. The Joint

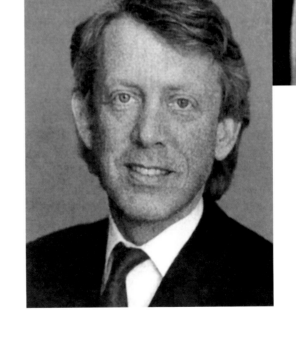

▲ *In 1994, two additional public members were added to the board: Charles H. (Pete) McTier, above, a foundation president in Atlanta, who is very knowledgeable on health issues; and Alexander M. Capron, below, a law professor at the University of Southern California and an expert in medical ethics and health policy.*

AGENDA • FOR • CHANGE
UPdATE

News from the Joint Commission

RECEIVED JUL 2 1 1992

The Agenda for Change

This first issue of the Joint Commission's *Update* represents an expansion of our efforts to keep you current concerning our Agenda for Change initiatives. This newsletter has been specifically designed to keep those who have expressed an interest in the Agenda for Change informed of our developmental activities and to provide rapid dissemination of our findings and implementation plans.

We plan to publish the newsletter three times each year. In this issue we cover a series of topics, including an overview of the Agenda for Change and our progress in the development of clinical and organizational indicators. Other articles describe plans for testing the new accreditation process in hospitals that have agreed to serve as pilot sites and the initiation of semi-annual invitational forums to coordinate the efforts of the Joint Commission and clinical specialty organizations. This issue also describes the composition of the Project Steering Committee and its role in these activities.

We intend to keep you fully informed of all major developments and findings of the Agenda for Change efforts. This is an ambitious and exciting project which we believe will greatly enhance our evaluation of the clinical and organizational performance of health care organizations. These efforts, however, will be successful only if we all work together. Your thoughts concerning the activities we describe in this newsletter are essential to this process. I encourage you to send us your comments, suggestions, and opinions concerning our current and proposed directions.

Please feel free to duplicate and distribute this newsletter as you wish. If you would like to suggest the addition of any individuals to our mailing list, please forward names and addresses to: *Department of Corporate Relations*, Joint Commission, 875 North Michigan Avenue, Suite 2200, Chicago, Illinois 60611.

We look forward to working with you.

Dennis S. O'Leary, MD
President

In the fall of 1986, the Joint Commission launched a major new developmental project entitled the Agenda for Change. The goal of the program is to develop an outcome-oriented monitoring and evaluation process that will assist health care organizations in improving the quality of the care they provide. As early as 1990, more than 5,000 hospitals accredited by the Joint Commission will initiate participation in the new monitoring, survey, and accreditation process. The more than 5,000 mental health centers, outpatient clinics, nursing homes, and hospices accredited by the Commission will begin the new process in 1991.

The new survey and accreditation process is the centerpiece of the Agenda for Change initiatives. Additional activities include:

• A communication effort to maintain and enhance Joint Commission relationships with provider organizations and health care professionals while fostering broader relationships with the government, business, labor, insurance, and consumer communities; and
• An education effort to expand and improve Joint Commission education and technical assistance services.

Task Forces Lay Groundwork For New Survey Process

Members of the Hospitalwide Clinical Indicators Task Force, the Obstetrical Care Task Force, the Anesthesia Care Task Force, and the Organization and Management Indicators Task Force have been appointed by the Joint Commission to begin the process of developing clinical and organizational indicators related to care in hospitals. The products of their efforts will form the foundation of the new performance-oriented accreditation system.

The Hospitalwide Clinical Indicators Task Force is led by James P. LoGerfo, MD, MPH. LoGerfo is Medical Director

(continued on page 2)

Why Initiate an Agenda for Change?

Because health care resources have become painfully finite and in view of the creation of altered payment incentives, quality of care has become a major public policy issue. When resources were abundant and quality was assumed to be inherent in the

(continued on page 2)

Volume 1, No. 1 • News about the Agenda for Change • September, 1987

(continued on page 2)

Agenda for Change Update *was published during the long implementation process of the original objectives outlined by the Agenda. This issue, from July 1992, explains the revision of the survey process that was underway at that time.*

began to do mid-cycle, random, unannounced surveys of 5 percent of accredited organizations. They were limited to the five performance areas that had been most problematic for each type of accredited organization in the previous year, and they did provide 16 to 24 hours advance notice to ensure that key personnel were present. In 1999, however, the board of commissioners approved the change to truly "unannounced" surveys in which no prior notice is given. Random, unannounced surveys responded to criticism that organizations often just put on a show for the Joint Commission, whose arrival was known well in advance, though they inevitably cast the Joint Commission as more of a regulator or inspector.

The revised standards and altered survey process together constituted a significant upgrading of quality. As had been the case historically, the revised standards and survey process drew upon professional opinion, including specialists in dozens of disciplines. They were the products of a collegial process that captured the best thinking of contemporary health care professionals. As had been true in the past, too, the revised standards and survey process manifested inherent tensions between the Joint Commission's educational, consultative, and evaluative roles. They also soon exposed tensions between serving its paying customers in health care organizations and serving the public, that is, the patients who use health care organizations.

Commission stepped up surveyor recruitment and training and endeavored to match surveyor qualifications more closely with the organizations they visited. The Joint Commission had long done focused surveys to follow up a serious problem that had been discovered during a routine survey visit and *for cause* surveys in response to a published or a privately communicated report of a serious failure or problem in a hospital. But in 1993, the Joint Commission

In the beginning, the response from the field to changes at the Joint Commission seemed quite favorable. A follow-up survey of hospital CEOs in 1990 showed a marked improvement in how they viewed Joint Commission performance over the prior year. Sixty percent indicated that the Joint Commission had improved its performance over the previous five years, compared to 38 percent in 1989. Only 9 percent believed its performance had worsened, compared to 26 percent in 1989. Survey-process evaluation questionnaires the Joint Commission conducted in 1991 were similarly positive and encouraging, particularly with respect to education and consultation. Around 1992, Raymond Scalettar, who consulted to the Joint Commission after leaving the board of commissioners, began to hear from hospital medical staffs that had recently had a survey and were enthusiastically implementing recommended changes. They had previously thought of the Joint Commission as punitive and they appreciated its new, more educational emphasis.

In 1993 and 1994, however, a negative reaction became manifest. One of the sorest points was cost. Survey fees for hospitals increased an average of 6 percent in 1992 and then another 6 percent in 1993, but certain large hospitals faced increases of up to 10 percent. (Nonhospital fees also rose, sometimes even more than hospital fees on a percentage basis.) On top of the annual increases, the board imposed a one-time, 6 percent special assessment on hospitals in 1992. It was collected between 1993 and 1995, at the time of the survey. Hospitals paid on average a special assessment of $1,100.

Fee increases and the special assessment underwrote the development and testing of the Indicator Measurement System (IMSystem), the outcomes data system the Joint Commission was developing. It was a multimillion-dollar undertaking that required careful testing before it could be launched. The complex system encountered significant technical difficulties and delays. The Joint Commission hoped to introduce IMSystem as an optional part of the accreditation process in 1996, but planned to make it a requirement eventually. Some hospital officials worried that they were being charged to give the Joint Commission

Although many hospital officials used to complain that the Joint Commission only looked at paperwork and process, and instead wanted it to look at outcomes, they started to become very nervous as outcomes measurement and dissemination actually approached.

sion education services and publications, about variations in surveyor performance, and about the rapid pace of change itself. In markets where hospitals were competing with each other, officials worried about the public release of organization-specific results. Would the Joint Commission soon be disseminating information that could materially hurt them? Although many hospital officials used to complain that the Joint Commission only looked at paperwork and process, and instead wanted it to look at outcomes, they started to become very nervous as outcomes measurement and dissemination actually approached.

The anxieties within hospitals about the Joint Commission were undoubtedly heightened by the rising level of anxiety within the health care industry more generally. By 1994, health care spending in the United States had reached $1 trillion, representing 14 percent of gross domestic product, by far the highest proportion of any economy in the world. At its best, the American health care system was outstanding. Advances in science and technology produced wonders and allowed lives to be saved. For many Americans, life expectancy and the quality of life had improved. But the system also had some great shortcomings, including 39 million Americans with no health insurance and another 20 million with inadequate health insurance. And the system was costly and inefficient. Businesses and government, which

a monopoly position, and that they would then be forced to pay it monopoly fees indefinitely.

Many hospital officials, particularly those in small and rural hospitals, worried about the indirect costs of complying with the revised standards and survey procedures. They complained about costs and about implied pressures to purchase Joint Commis-

together paid most of the bill, were starting to resist annual increases in premiums that exceeded every other category of spending. Hospitals, which received the largest single piece of the health care dollar, were under pressure from payers to reduce their bills. Diagnostic-Related Groups (DRGs), through which the government reimbursed hospitals, were well established, and prospective payment contracts and capitated systems were growing in importance. Hospital competition, closings, consolidations, and health networks were all rising.

In 1993, recently elected U.S. president Bill Clinton put his wife, Hillary, a lawyer and children's advocate, in charge of developing legislation to address major problems in the health care system. There were lengthy, secretive deliberations, extensive public outreach and discussion, and delays necessitated by higher priority action on the budget and the new administration's economic program. But in September, the Clintons introduced the Health Security Act with a public relations blitz. It was a very long and complex piece of legislation that was built around managed competition, regional health alliances, and government mandates and incentives. AMA and AHA leaders were consulted during the plan's gestation, but their suggestions had been ignored. The two associations dreaded federal regulation and controls and worried about HMOs, all of which were certain to expand under the Clinton plan.

Both associations were nervous about becoming too publicly involved in the controversy that followed the plan's introduction, however.

Ideologically conservative Republicans, indemnity health insurers and pharmaceutical manufacturers did not shy away from the controversy — they fanned the flames. The Health Insurance Association of America sponsored notoriously effective television commercials featuring "Harry and Louise," which appealed to the large number of people who were content with the status quo and fearful of government bureaucracy. The Clinton administration rejected a more modest plan offered by Jim Cooper, a Tennessee Democrat. Moreover, the Clinton administration failed to build the kind of bipartisan support that would have been necessary for its plan to prevail. Some believed it was flawed because it was too ambitious, while others thought it had not gone far enough, failing to propose universal, government-sponsored coverage. Stalled in committee or multiple committees, the legislation never even came to a vote on the House or Senate floors.

It is worth summarizing what has happened since the attempt to enact broad reform of the health care system in 1994. Ironically, some of the things that doctors and hospitals had feared about the Clinton plan, namely the expansion of managed care and of federal control, have come to pass anyway. Unfortunately, the number of uninsured and underinsured

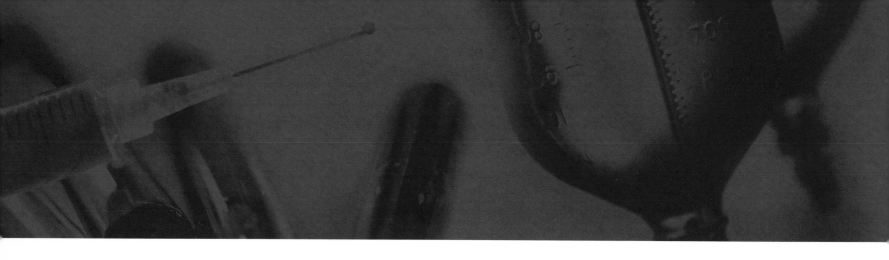

people has also increased slightly. Price resistance from private payers, specifically large employers, and from public payers, especially through bipartisan efforts that balanced the federal budget, halted the growth in the health care sector's relative share of the domestic economy. Overall health care spending has been essentially flat since that time. Health care organizations have been buffeted by market and government forces, and the Joint Commission has been whipsawed in turn. For example, spending reductions under the Balanced Budget Act of 1997 led to a 45 percent reduction in federal payments for home care over two years, and that in turn forced many home care organizations to drop accreditation. Lesser reductions in government payments for hospital and long-term care have also recently caused reductions in accreditation programs in those areas as well, though not as great as in home care. "Chaotic" is probably the word most frequently used by insiders to describe the health care system in which they work today.

With its ambitious and multi-faceted program of change, the Joint Commission was, in a certain sense, riding down a parallel track to the Clinton administration in 1993 and 1994. It was attempting to implement a major restructuring of standards and the survey process that was both expensive and anxiety-provoking for its paying customers. Hospitals continued to complain about the cost and conduct of surveys

and about the Joint Commission's becoming too regulatory. A number of state hospital associations began to talk about actually dropping accreditation and obtaining deemed status through other means, including state inspection, for which they did not have to pay. However, most hospital officials still strongly preferred a voluntary system of accreditation to government inspection and licensure. The Joint Commission's annual opinion survey of hospital CEOs in 1994 was actually very favorable about the new standards and survey process and even about the Joint Commission's overall performance, though 25 percent of respondents were somewhat or very dissatisfied.

In response to complaints, criticisms and anxieties that were surfacing in the field and at board meetings, O'Leary, board members and representatives of the Joint Commission held a series of "town hall" meetings with state hospital associations around the country. In response to these meetings, O'Leary organized a work group on small and rural hospitals, which were under the greatest financial pressure. All nine AHA regions were represented on this group and non-accredited as well as accredited hospitals. Individuals were chosen *because* they were outspoken, recalls Tommy Mullins, a member of the group and a veteran hospital administrator from Madison, West Virginia. The first meeting in October 1994, which was scheduled to last a half-day, went on for practically a full day, with the participation of

> "Chaotic" is probably the word most frequently used by insiders to describe the health care system in which they work today.

Joint Commission staff and four board members, including the incumbent and incoming chairman.

Perspectives reported that members "wasted little time in identifying core concerns: financial constraints, including 'hard' and 'soft' costs of complying with onerous regulations imposed by external entities that do not understand the realities of providing care in a rural environment. In addition, participants underlined the difficult choices they must make when allocating resources, expressed disdain for the 'bigger is better' prejudice of large purchasers and emphasized the competitive pressures they faced from acquisitive health care organizations." The work group delineated eight key issues that were to be the focus for collaborative problem-solving over the following six to twelve months.

A CRISIS OF CONFIDENCE AND ITS AFTERMATH

Members of this work group, board members and AHA commissioners, including D. Kirk Oglesby Jr., who was chairman of the Joint Commission, were surprised by an AHA press conference held in Chicago on December 8, 1994. The AHA board of trustees released a statement that began with an assertion of strong support for the Joint Commission and for accreditation as the most appropriate vehicle for assuring the public about the quality of the nation's hospitals and health systems. "Regrettably," the statement continued, "after more than a year of

study and discussion with the field through the AHA's regional policy boards, with state and metropolitan hospital associations, and other Joint Commission sponsors, the Board has concluded that there today is a crisis in confidence in the Joint Commission and that immediate and substantive change is necessary." The crisis was "the result of the cumulative impact of chronic performance problems, marketing of too many add-on services and a fundamental lack of responsiveness to the needs of hospitals and their medical staffs. While leadership of the Joint Commission has tried to address some of these issues, the response has been uneven and untimely." The statement called for a meeting of the sponsoring organizations within 30 days to "institute immediate action to rectify these issues and to begin discussion about strategic planning for the future of the Joint Commission."

A sizeable number of reporters from the trade and general press participated in the press conference, either in person or by telephone. The AHA was represented by Dick Davidson, president, Carolyn Roberts, chairperson, and Jack Lord, a senior adviser for clinical affairs. In her opening statement, Roberts began by stressing the AHA's continued support for the Joint Commission, but then focused on various concerns: costs, communications, surveyor quality, "relentless marketing of education programs, publications and other products." The intent of the AHA board's action

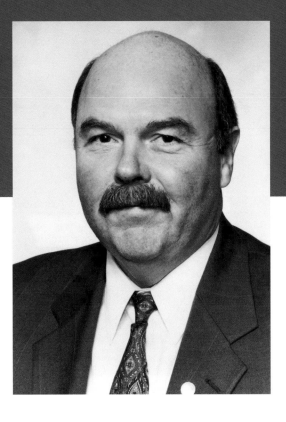

was to set a process in motion to remedy "today's operational problems" and then to plan for the Joint Commission's long-term future. Roberts pointed out that hospitals accounted for about 71 percent of the Joint Commission's $115 million budget.

Davidson said that there were between 15 and 20 states that were currently looking at alternatives to Joint Commission accreditation. "And if in fact we saw a desertion of a substantial number of our members away from the Joint Commission we could see a potential collapse."

Davidson also noted the shift of the Joint Commission's role from educational to regulatory. "Now they're moving into another role as voice to the public with regard to performance standards and accountability," Davidson observed. His preference was that the Joint Commission "go back to its roots of just helping institutions improve their performance." When Davidson and Roberts were asked

whether public disclosure of performance reports had anything to do with the current crisis of confidence, they denied that it did and said that the AHA fully supported disclosure.

Critical resolutions regarding the Joint Commission had periodically been passed at the annual meetings of the AMA and the AHA. Indeed, the AMA House of Delegates, meeting in Honolulu at practically the same time as the AHA board, coincidentally approved by voice vote a resolution that called for evaluating the implications of withdrawing from the Joint Commission and looking at alternatives. This resolution had been engineered by the AMA's Hospital Medical Staff Section, which had been concerned over the costs and benefits of accreditation. Its concerns had been exacerbated by perceived dilution of medical staff authority in the *1995 Accreditation Manual for Hospitals*.

Over the years, one corporate member or another had said unflattering things about the Joint Commission to the press. But a corporate member had never before called a press conference to attack the Joint Commission like this. "Isn't this fairly drastic to go from closed door sessions to calling a press conference?" asked David Burda, a veteran reporter for *Modern Healthcare*. Davidson responded that "these signals have been sent time and time again. Sometimes you have to send the signal in a different way to be sure that it's really going to be paid attention to."

In his published account, Burda stressed the AHA ultimatum, passing over any mention of its assertion of support for accreditation, perhaps because he did not find it convincing. He also gave almost equal attention to the AMA's possible withdrawal.

In a more comprehensive account in *American Medical News*, Linda Oberman quoted the soothing words of William E. Jacott, the head of the AMA delegation to the Joint Commission. "We need to be constructive," said Jacott. "It is not our desire to scuttle the commission." Jacott predicted that the AMA eventually might accredit physicians, but expected that the Joint Commission would handle broader accreditation and that the AMA would continue to participate on its board. (The AMA subsequently started a physicians' accreditation program, but after investing $12 million, it terminated the program in early 2000.) Oberman also noted that Public Citizen, an organization founded by consumer advocate Ralph Nader, questioned whether relying on a private accrediting organization for a public regulatory function was in the public interest. An attorney for Public Citizen labeled the Joint Commission's recent release of hospital accreditation data a "public relations ploy," for the commission was charging $30 for each performance report and was providing organizations the names of those who requested data on them. Moreover, she asserted that provider governance of the commission com-

promised the data to begin with.

The press conference angered some board members who felt they had been blindsided. They liken it to the surprise attack on Pearl Harbor or to D-Day. "It was painful for me personally," recalls Oglesby, who had been on the board of commissioners from 1989 to 1991 and who had then returned at the AHA's request specifically to serve as Joint Commission chairman. "You don't like to be in a combative environment," says Oglesby, who has loyally served both the AHA and the Joint Commission. "I thought it was a dirty trick on the part of the AHA," notes William W. Kridelbaugh, an ACS commissioner, who succeeded Oglesby as chairman in January 1995. "When the AHA came along with this bludgeon of a press conference in December, I thought we were in really serious trouble. I had supposed that

> Over the years, one corporate member or another had said unflattering things about the Joint Commission to the press. But a corporate member had never before called a press conference to attack the Joint Commission like this.

all of the AHA commissioners knew about this. Later on I found out that maybe they didn't."

In a written response to state hospital association officials, the Joint Commission expressed its surprise and disappointment that the AHA had chosen to raise its concerns in a press conference rather than directly. Contradicting Davidson, the statement noted that during the past year it had "received no direct communication from the AHA leadership about its 'growing number of concerns.'" It recognized that the changes in the accreditation process had come at a particularly stressful time for health care organizations in general and hospitals in particular. Although the Agenda for Change had required a significant investment, its funding over the previous several years had been constrained and had "followed a strategy suggested by an AHA panel of financial advisers in 1992." According to the Joint Commission's statement, the proportion of hospitals' operating expenses that went to survey fees had not changed since 1988, a mere 0.01 percent.

The Joint Commission statement noted that an independent survey of hospitals in 1994 indicated that more than 80 percent found the new survey process to be "more interactive, consultative and valuable than previous surveys." It also reported that the number of focused surveys for hospitals had actually fallen to 1,450 in 1994 from 5,000 in 1989. The Joint Commission statement described a number of other

recent initiatives and it asserted the Joint Commission's financial health. The Joint Commission accredited more than 11,000 organizations of various kinds, and it accredited more hospitals than the total membership of the AHA, according to the statement.

As the AHA had requested and as the by-laws provided, a meeting of the corporate members was held to discuss AHA concerns on January 9, 1995. Less than two weeks later, the regular meeting of the board was devoted largely to AHA concerns. These were tense meetings. Although the substantive issues were important, it was also fairly obvious that the AHA wanted to oust O'Leary. In a private meeting with Kridelbaugh in early January, an AHA representative predicted that O'Leary would be gone soon and there were rumors about who Dick Davidson wanted to place in the job. Following the press conference and for the better part of the year, pressures were intense and morale at the Joint Commission was low.

In the early months of the crisis, O'Leary considered resigning for the good of the organization. However, other staff members, friends, board officers, and O'Leary himself concluded that it would be more damaging to the Joint Commission if he were to resign. At the suggestion of a consultant and friend who worried about possible damage to O'Leary's reputation from the ongoing debate, O'Leary hired outside counsel from a prominent firm. The attorney's silent observation of several meetings during the cri-

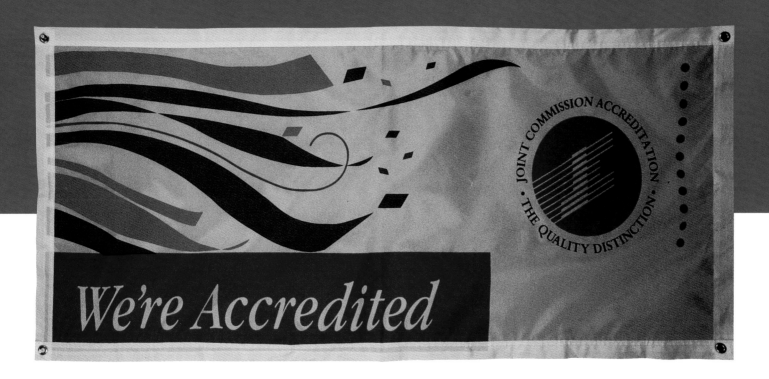

sis sent a signal to the AHA's leaders that O'Leary was "playing for keeps" and would not fold his tent.

The political situation was reminiscent of the attempted removal of John Affeldt, though the AHA was isolated this time — it did not have the AMA as a co-conspirator. As the recent voice vote by the AMA House of Delegates indicated, there was certainly dissatisfaction with the Joint Commission within AMA ranks, but Bill Jacott, who led the AMA delegation, had a high regard for O'Leary. In addition, he believed in working from within. Moreover, the seven public members of the board, including the at-large nurse representative, supported O'Leary, as did the colleges and the ADA. The AHA did not have the votes to topple O'Leary, and its heavy-handed tactics only hurt its position.

In his statements to the board and the public, O'Leary corrected some factual errors by the AHA. He also expressed a strong perceptual difference, for he believed that although none of the current furor was *ostensibly* about public disclosure of performance reports, anxieties about them were actually fundamental to the furor. "When credible performance information flows into the public domain," O'Leary wrote in the first issue of *Perspectives* in 1995, "the implications can be profound." Yet O'Leary also acknowledged operational problems and shortcomings at the Joint Commission itself. Jacott observes that, to O'Leary's credit, "he was quick to respond with an action plan that was clearly laid out and was a dynamic and not a static document." In his *Perspectives* column, O'Leary recalled that prior to accepting the presidency 10 years before, he himself had not been a happy or a quiet customer of the Joint Commission. "Notwithstanding the substantial progress since made, you who remain in the field still hold an IOU for not-yet-finished deliverables," he humbly wrote. "With the Board of Commissioners' endorsement at its January meeting, the Joint Commission now has a specific Action Plan to satisfy that IOU."

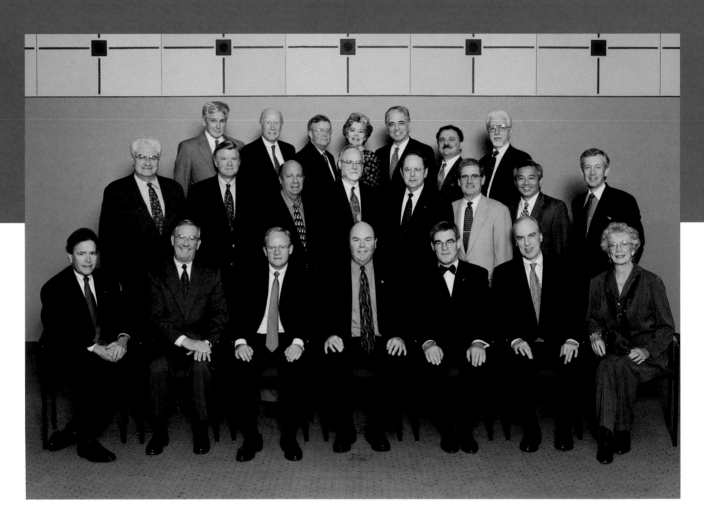

The Action Plan included measurable performance objectives and timelines. They related to staff responsiveness; re-engineering of the survey process; and surveyor credibility, monitoring, and performance. John Castle recalls that the AHA's overwhelming focus during the crisis was not on management performance, however, but on cutting prices. It definitely scored some successes in that respect. The board imposed an immediate price freeze on fees charged for regular full surveys. It instituted a substantial reduction in the number of focused surveys and stopped charging for them, meaning that the Joint Commission had to absorb their cost. Those decisions reduced revenues while increasing expenses. With black ink steadily turning red, the budget had to be redone sev-

eral times over the next year. There was a freeze on pay raises and rounds of lay-offs. "It was a terrible time," recalls a senior staff member sadly.

In the Action Plan, the Joint Commission agreed to limit changes in standards to important issues that clearly related to quality patient care. It promised to accelerate a project aimed at simplifying the language in the standards manual and it authorized testing of a pilot project for improving the accreditation process that had been developed by the work group of small and rural hospitals. Accordingly, the Orion Project, involving a continuous accreditation process on a regional level, was launched in the spring.

The idea of continuous accreditation is very much alive today. In fact, continuous accreditation is a focus of a major initiative of the Joint Commission, commencing in 2000, called the Accreditation Process Improvement (API) project. Headed by Executive Vice President of accreditation operations Russell Massaro, API is intended to increase the real and perceived value of accreditation to accredited organizations, deeming authorities and purchasers, and the lay public. Two characteristics of the new process are periodic reporting of performance measurement results by health care organizations and (yet to be approved by the board) an on-site survey every 18 months.

Meanwhile, the concerns of the Hospital Medical Staff Section of the AMA were addressed by a work group that the Joint Commission convened in the summer of 1994 and that included AMA representatives. It had come up with changes in the offending standards to reemphasize medical staff authority in improving the quality of care.

In what was probably the most important concession to its customers, however, the Joint Commission surrendered any notion of monopolizing performance measurement. It agreed to "re-configuration of the IMSystem to utilize measures and measurement systems developed by other entities, with the long-term objectives of offering a varied menu of relevant measures to all types of organizations as part of the accreditation process." There were many not-for-profit and for-profit entities that had entered or were contemplating entering the performance measurement field in health care. In February, the Joint Commission wrote letters to 250 of them, inviting collaboration, and an independent Council on Performance Measurement was created to evaluate prospective measurement systems. Moreover, the Joint Commission began to contemplate selling IMSystem to a private vendor.

The Action Plan met many of the concerns that the AHA had expressed, but it did not completely end the sense of crisis or unpleasantness either at the staff or board levels. Over the next two years, the performance of O'Leary and the staff were closely monitored, as were opinion surveys from the field. Interpretations of survey findings were debated at board meetings. In *Perspectives*, the Joint Commission trumpeted its progress, successes, and innovations.

Meanwhile, a board task force on corporate governance came up empty. Although AHA leaders had at the outset talked about wanting to address long-term strategic issues once short-term operational problems were resolved, its overriding interests struck some as short-term and financial. Father Byron recalls speaking one year in support of the AHA position against a survey fee increase. After the board voted against the increase, the AHA put out a press release taking full credit for stopping the increase, ignoring the importance of the board structure in its efforts to appease its own members.

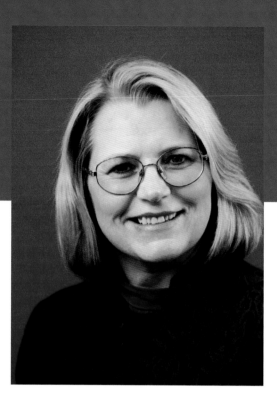

In early 1996, John Castle, who had become Joint Commission treasurer and was in line to become the first public member to serve as chairman, resigned from the board. A very active businessman, Castle made a considerable sacrifice to serve on the board but felt that much of his time was being wasted. "It was really a continuation of the crisis that made me leave," Castle reflects. "It was a series of requests that came out of the AHA that were obviously not constructive. I had no axe to grind. I viewed myself as a representative of the American public. I wanted an organization that did a more effective job in accreditation to enhance the performance of hospitals."

Dean Morton succeeded Castle as treasurer. In September 1996, Morton proposed the 1997 budget, which included a total of $2 million in survey fee increases, representing a 2 percent fee increase for the hospital program and larger increases for other programs. O'Leary pointed out that the budget had been developed within the context of objectives that had

been previously approved by the board, including an emphasis on core activities and investments in the future. To O'Leary's dismay, the AHA now vigorously challenged the budget within the board. In the ensuing debate, the AHA largely got its way — the increase in hospital survey fees was rescinded. So for the third straight year, there was no increase. The only such increase that survived the budget debate was one for the network accreditation program. Like Castle, Morton preferred not wasting his time. After he left the meeting, he too resigned from the board.

Over time, however, the crisis atmosphere of 1994-1995 gradually receded, though there are occasional reverberations. In 1997, Bernard L. Hengesbaugh and Gerald M. Shea succeeded Castle and Morton as public members. Hengesbaugh, a senior executive with CNA Insurance Companies when he joined the board, became CNA's chairman and CEO in 1999. Shea is assistant to the president for governmental affairs at the AFL-CIO. He also serves on the federal Medicare Payment Advisory Committee. In 1995, James R. Tallon Jr. had taken Carolyn Lewis's place. (Lewis joined the AHA board, which she now chairs.) A veteran state legislator and legislative leader in New York, Tallon has been president of the United Hospital Fund of New York since 1993. In 1998, Father Lawrence Biondi, a Jesuit priest, linguist, and president of Saint Louis University, succeeded Father Byron.

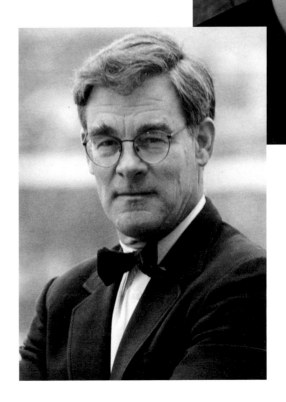

The new public members, like the remaining ones, brought diverse perspectives and experience to the table. They helped ensure that the Joint Commission was responsive to the broader public interest. They have been a considerable force for expanding and improving public disclosure and expanding communications with the public. The Joint Commission has become much more accessible to the public than it ever was before. Performance reports on all accredited organizations are provided free of charge on the Joint Commission's Web site. As always, it is a working board and a very hard-working one at that. It is reportedly more cohesive than it was. However, John Helfrick and Bill Jacott, the board's chairmen from 1997 to 2000, were unable to obtain voting privileges for public members on by-law changes. It is not out of the question yet, for the AHA has public membership on its board and the AMA house of delegates has voted to add a non-physician member to its board of trustees.

The implementation of performance measurement was slowed down a little by hospital objections in 1995. The Joint Commission did sell the IMSystem to a private vendor, which eliminated the possibility that it was seeking to monopolize this area. However, the Joint Commission remained fully committed to the principle of performance measurement. In 1997, it launched the ambitious ORYX initiative, aimed at bringing outcomes and other performance measures

▲ *Board member John Helfrick (above), wrote a letter to the entire board expressing his concerns about patient safety issues that were in the headlines in 1995. Helfrick served as the sole American Dental Association representative on the board from 1992 to 1999 and was board chairman in 1997 and 1998. John Noble (below), also a board member, has chaired the Codman Award Selection Committee since its inception.*

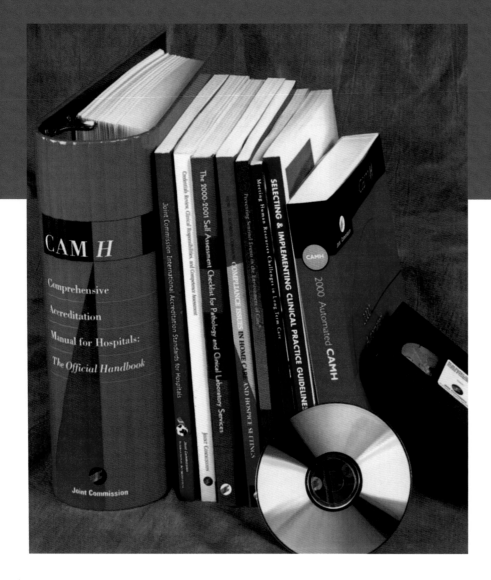

improve organization performance. Appropriately enough the awards were named in honor of Ernest A. Codman, whose groundbreaking book, *A Study in Hospital Efficiency*, the Joint Commission reprinted in 1996, helping to rehabilitate his memory. By disseminating information about the Codman Award winners and their accomplishments and successes, the Joint Commission helps educate and inspire the field. John Noble, a board member, has chaired the Codman Award Selection Committee since its inception. In another educational initiative, the Joint Commission in 1997 collaborated with five universities in establishing the Academy for Healthcare Quality, for post-graduate continuing education. Unfortunately, this "university without walls" was a good idea, but not economically feasible and was dissolved two years later.

Sporadically throughout its history, the Joint Commission had been involved in accrediting hospitals outside the United States as well as international consulting. In the late 1990s, the board formally recognized a growing demand for accreditation internationally, and an even larger potential for providing consultation and educational services around the world. In 1997, it established Joint Commission Resources (JCR) as a successor to Quality Health Resources, its consulting subsidiary, with Tina Donahue as its CEO. In 1999, Donahue was succeeded by Karen Timmons when plans were made to expand

to the accreditation process in all accreditation programs. Today organizations are required to report outcomes from indicators they have selected. In the near future, organizations will be required to begin reporting on preselected core measures.

To bolster its educational mission and balance its regulatory activities, the Joint Commission made three big investments in the late 1990s. In 1997, it began to give awards to recognize outstanding achievement by health care organizations and individuals in the use of performance measurement to

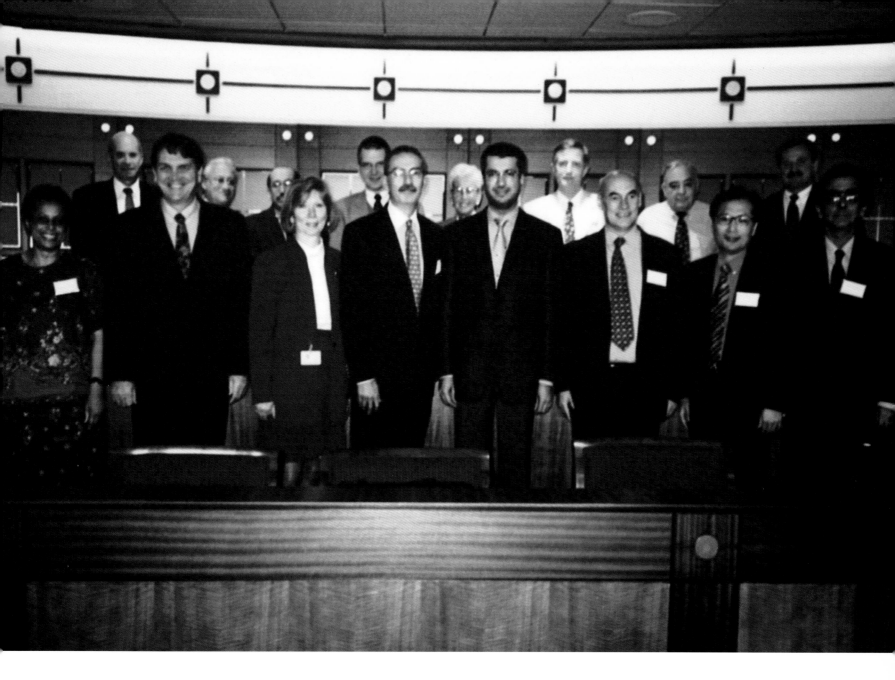

▲ Shown here is the International Accreditation Principles and Standards Development Task Force that developed the first set of international hospital standards in 1998. From left to right are Maureen Wellington (Zimbabwe), Clive B. Ross (New Zealand), Stuart Whittaker (South Africa), Willes B. Goldbech (USA), Saled M. Almulla (United Arab Emirates), Tina Donahue (Joint Commission Resources), David Marx (Czech Republic), Paul vanOstenberg (Joint Commission Resources), Margaretta Styles (USA), Yazed A. Ohaly (Saudi Arabia), Rafal Nizankowski (Poland), Lluis Bohigas (Spain), Rodolpho A. Armas-Merino (Chile), Ping Huang (Republic of China), James Janeski (Joint Commission Resources), and Jose Noronha (Brazil). Not pictured are Charles Shaw (United Kingdom), Nick Klayenga (The Netherlands), and Christopher Straub (Germany).

> Horrific incidents in accredited hospitals in a number of cities, including Boston, New York, and Tampa, were featured news stories that drew the public's attention.

JCR to include all Joint Commission education, publication, and continuous survey readiness (CSR) activities. The new organization established the first set of international standards for health care ever developed, but they were consistent with principles that had been developed by the International Society for Quality in Health Care, of which the Joint Commission had been a charter member. International accreditation of hospitals under the Joint Commission standards was initiated in Spain in 1998 under a partnership with the Avedis Donabedian Foundation. Hospital General de Catalunya was the first to be accredited. In December 1999 the first accreditation survey under the new international standards resulted in the Joint Commission International accreditation of Hospital Isrealita Albert Einstein, a private, non-profit, 410-bed hospital in São Paulo, Brazil. Only the future will tell how successful the Joint Commission's international endeavors will be.

NEW SPOTLIGHT ON SAFETY

In recent years, as a result of academic studies and highly publicized incidents of hospital error, patient safety has moved to the forefront. In 1991, Troyen Brennan, Lucian Leape, and others reported in the *New England Journal of Medicine* on the results of the Harvard Medical Practice Study. On the basis of a review of about 30,000 randomly selected records of patients hospitalized in New York State in 1984, these researchers determined that adverse events occurred in 4 percent of hospitalizations and that 14 percent of these events were fatal. In a dramatic illustration of the problem's scale, the authors extrapolated that as many people were dying from preventable deaths in American hospitals as would die if three jumbo jets crashed every two days.

Horrific incidents in accredited hospitals in a number of cities, including Boston, New York, and Tampa, were featured news stories that drew the public's attention. Preventable adverse events in hospitals, such as amputation of the wrong leg, deaths from medication errors and some suicides, obviously raised questions with the public about the value of the "seal of approval" connoted by accreditation. What did these horrible errors say about accreditation? What did they say about the Joint Commission? What did they say about health care in the United States?

Concerned about these important questions, John Helfrick, a board member, wrote a letter to the

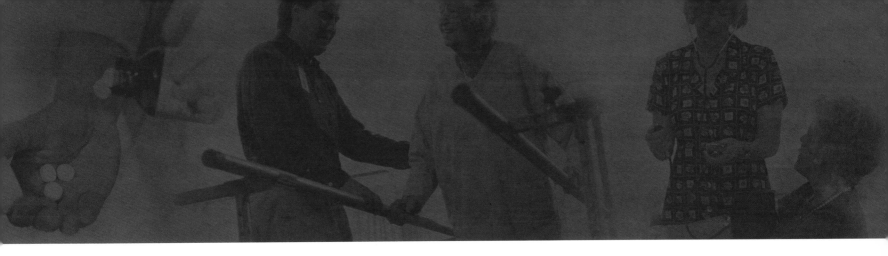

entire board recommending that the Joint Commission become more involved in patient safety issues. In response, the Joint Commission began in early 1996 to formulate specific policies on sentinel events, defined as serious undesirable occurrences that result in the loss of patient life, limb, or function. When the Joint Commission was made aware of a possible sentinel event, it conducted an unannounced survey. The policy contemplated that if it was determined that the organization had substantial control over the circumstances that led to the event, the organization would be given conditional accreditation pending the completion of an acceptable analysis of the event focused on reducing the risk of similar events occurring in the future. Subsequently, instead of conditional accreditation, "accreditation watch" was established as the designation for organizations that had experienced certain defined sentinel events pending completion of such an analysis. This change was announced in October 1996, during the Annenberg Conference, a multidisciplinary conference on examining and preventing errors in health care held by the Joint Commission and three other organizations at the Annenberg Center for Health Sciences in California.

Board leaders and staff soon came to believe, however, that their initial approach to sentinel events was essentially punitive and was unlikely to be effective. "The blame and punishment approach we were using

was getting us nowhere," Helfrick, who was board chairman in 1997 and 1998, recalls. It depended on learning about errors from third sources or from hospitals, which were then "rewarded" for reporting themselves by being placed on "Accreditation Watch." The academic research suggested that many more errors occurred than were ever likely going to be reported. Following protracted debates in 1997, the board decided on the concept of encouraging organizations to report sentinel events and the findings of their root cause analyses of those events.

From the reports and "root cause" analyses, the Joint Commission looked for common patterns of errors in order to inform and educate the field. As many experts have argued, errors are usually the result of poor processes, not of incompetent or inattentive people or, more rarely, of malicious professionals or impostors. The reporting program had worthwhile results. For example, the data showed that potassium chloride came in vials that closely resembled sterile saline and other commonly used injectable medications and was, upon occasion, mistakenly injected intravenously in concentrated form — a process error that resulted in a significant number of accidental deaths. After the Joint Commission issued a sentinel event alert to the field explaining how such accidents could be prevented, the frequency with which they were reported or otherwise brought to the attention of the Joint Commission fell dramatically. Following dissemination of sentinel event alerts, there have also been reductions in the frequency of reports to the Joint Commission of accidental deaths from restraints, inpatient suicides and infant abductions.

Both the AHA and the AMA were nervous about their members having to report sentinel event data because reports might be discoverable in legal proceedings. Since there is still a vast discrepancy between the number of reported adverse events and the number estimated by academic researchers, it is reasonable to conclude that substantial underreporting of sentinel or adverse events exists today. Educating Congress and the executive branch on the need for a federal and preemptive statute therefore has been a focus of the Joint Commission's Washington office. It succeeded in getting such a bill passed in the House of Representatives in 1998. (Established in 1993, this small but very active office has been directed from the beginning by Margaret VanAmringe, a former program director with HCFA.) In a change directed at underscoring the importance of patient safety and the need to pursue it ceaselessly, the board approved a change in the wording of the mission statement in October 1999: (new words are italicized) "The mission...is to *continuously* improve the *safety and* quality of care provided to the public...."

Then, at the end of November 1999, *To Err Is Human,* a report from the prestigious Institute of Medicine, received wide public attention. Extrapolating from the 1991 Harvard study and several more recent ones, the report estimated that anywhere from 44,000 to 98,000 Americans die each year because of medical errors in hospitals. If even the lower estimate was correct, more people die from medical errors than from motor vehicle accidents, breast cancer or AIDS. Medication errors alone were estimated to cause more than 7,000 deaths annually. William C. Richardson, the panel's chairman, said, "these stunningly high rates of medical errors...are simply unacceptable in a medical system that promises first to 'do no harm.'" The panel called for a new federal agency to monitor patient safety and for mandatory reporting of errors. Its recommendations received President Clinton's endorsement and some administrative action, but full implementation will require congressional action.

Not surprisingly, the most spirited debate within the 19-member Institute of Medicine panel revolved around issues of confidentiality versus the patient's right to know. "If the treatment results in injury, the patient has the right to know," Lucian Leape, a panel member, reflected to a reporter afterward. "The fact that doctors are scared about getting sued for that is unfortunate. But it doesn't mean we ought to eliminate the ethical imperative." Others, however, pointed out that the liability climate discouraged open discussion and reporting of mistakes. Leape himself has often spoken out strongly against a "blame and punishment" approach to errors, instead of taking a systems and process approach.

The Office of Inspector General (OIG) also issued an important report in 1999, *The External Review of Hospital Quality*. This lengthy report focused on the roles played by the Joint Commission and the state agencies in reviewing hospitals and by HCFA in overseeing these bodies. It called for HCFA to hold the Joint Commission and state agencies more accountable for their performance, though it recommended that HCFA should seek a balance between collegial and regulatory modes of oversight. The OIG report noted that Joint Commission surveys were "unlikely to detect substandard patterns of care or individual practitioners with questionable skills." Responding promptly to the OIG report, the Joint Commission's board strengthened the integrity of the survey process, including the establishment of truly unannounced random surveys.

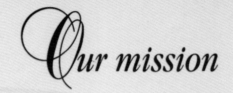

ur mission

is to continuously improve the

safety and quality of care provided to the

public through the provision of

health care accreditation and

related services that support performance

improvement in health care

organizations.

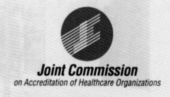

Joint Commission
on Accreditation of Healthcare Organizations

▲ **The Joint Commission adopted this updated mission statement in October 1999.**

Epilogue

As this book goes to press, the Joint Commission has undertaken significant revisions of its accreditation process as well as a study of its management and governance structures. Questions that are being asked today both within the Joint Commission and outside it are not entirely new. Are surveyors to be inspectors or teachers or both? How should quality be defined and by whom? What is the proper balance between capabilities and performance in organizational standards? Does a voluntary, collegial method of oversight work as well as, equal to, or better than a mandatory, directive one? To what extent should the public and the government depend on the Joint Commission, a private organization, to carry out a public responsibility? How and to what extent should the public be involved in the accreditation process and in governance and oversight of the body that determines accreditation? What is the most appropriate way to pay for accreditation and who should serve on the Joint Commission's board and on the committees that set standards and make accreditation decisions?

During its first 50 years, the Joint Commission has developed answers to these questions. The answers are reflected in the complex operations, standards, procedures, and governance that the Joint Commission has today. During these 50 years, the Joint Commission has not operated in a vacuum. It has had to respond to both external and internal pressures. As a result of these pressures, there is much greater public representation and public accountability today than there was in 1951. There is much greater emphasis on organizational performance as opposed to organizational capabilities than there was 50 years ago. On the other hand, the balance between surveyors as inspectors and surveyors as teachers has been in a constant state of flux, as has the balance between collegial and mandatory oversight. A fundamental change in financing accreditation was put into place in 1964, though there has been constant modification in the details of financing ever since.

The past strongly suggests that change will continue to occur, though only time will tell what will change and what will remain the same and to what effect. A constant throughout these 50 years, and during the four preceding decades when the American College of Surgeons first developed a certification program, has been the overarching purpose of improving the quality of health care provided to the public, first in hospitals and then in various other organized settings as well. Whatever happens in the future, it is to be hoped that this high purpose will endure both in principle and in practice.

Acknowledgments

The author and the Joint Commission would like to thank the Joint Commission's 50th Anniversary Celebration Committee for their guidance on and review of the manuscript for this book. Members of the committee are: James W. Holsinger Jr., MD (Chairman); Lawrence Biondi, SJ; Rufus K. Broadaway, MD; William J. Byron, SJ; Daniel S. Ellis, MD; Timothy T. Flaherty, MD; Irwin N. Frank, MD; Elbert E. Gilbertson; Mary T. Herald, MD; William E. Jacott, MD; M. J. Jurkiewicz, MD; Charles A. McCallum, DMD, MD; Charles H. McTier; John Noble, MD; and Carolyn C. Roberts.

We would like to thank the following who graciously agreed to be interviewed for this history: John E. Affeldt, MD; Donald Avant; Paul B. Batalden, MD; Harold Bressler, JD; Rufus K. Broadaway, MD; William J. Byron, SJ; Jean Gayton Carroll; John K. Castle; Mary Cesare Murphy; Barbara Donaho, RN; Daniel S. Ellis, MD; Leo Gehrig, MD; Elbert E. Gilbertson; C. Rollins Hanlon, MD; John F. Helfrick, DDS; Harry Hinton; Charles M. Jacobs; William E. Jacott, MD; William F. Jessee, MD; M. J. Jurkiewicz, MD, DDS; William W. Kridelbaugh, MD; Carolyn B. Lewis; Charles A. McCallum, DMD, MD; Barbara A. McCann; J. Alexander McMahon; John Milton; Robert H. Moser, MD; Tommy H. Mullins; Alan Nelson, MD; Duncan Neuhauser, PhD; D. Kirk Oglesby Jr.; Dennis O'Leary, MD; Carole Patterson, RN; Laura Reeder; Bruce Roberts, JD; James S. Roberts, MD; Judith A. Ryan, PhD, RN; James Sammons, MD; Sally Ann Sample, RN, MN; Raymond Scalettar, MD; Paul M. Schyve, MD; James Simon, JD; Rosemary A. Stevens, PhD; Mary Tellis-Nayak, RN; Karen H. Timmons; Margaret VanAmringe; Eleanor Wagner; and John H. Westerman.

We would also like to acknowledge the assistance of Janet Aleccia, Laura Shedore, Laura Reeder, and Mack Dieden, in compiling archival publications, documents, photos, and other research materials. Thank you to Barbara Hone, library administrator at the American College of Surgeons, and to Information Specialist Sara Beazley and Eloise C. Foster, director of the American Hospital Association Resource Center, for their invaluable assistance in locating archival photographs for this book. Thank you to William Bullerman for designing the color overlay on this book cover. We would like to thank the following who reviewed the manuscript: Cathy Barry Ipema; Dennis S. O'Leary, MD; Laura Reeder; James S. Roberts, MD; Paul M. Schyve, MD; Karen H. Timmons; and Eleanor Wagner.

Finally, the author gratefully acknowledges the assistance of Frances Perveiler, his liaison at the Joint Commission. He enjoyed working with Fran immensely.

1847 The American Medical Association (AMA) is established.

1869 Ernest A. Codman is born in Boston to a prosperous Brahmin family.

1895 Frederick Winslow Taylor publishes his first paper on scientific management, which applies rational principles to industrial processes and is aimed at optimizing efficiency.

Ernest A. Codman graduates from Harvard Medical School.

1899 Association of Hospital Superintendents is founded. It changes its name in 1908 to the American Hospital Association (AHA).

1910 Clinical Congress of Surgeons is formed with its first meeting in Chicago; subsequent meetings are held in Philadelphia in 1911 and New York in 1912.

Publication of the Flexner report on medical education, by Abraham Flexner of the Carnegie Foundation, symbolizes a key moment in professional reform.

Ernest Codman proposes the "end result system of hospital standardization." Under this system, a hospital would track every patient it treated long enough to determine whether the treatment was effective. If the treatment was not effective, the hospital would then attempt to determine why, so that similar cases could be treated successfully in the future.

1911 Ernest A. Codman opens a 20-bed proprietary hospital that is organized around the End Result Idea and begins methodically documenting its activities.

1912 New York Clinical Congress of Surgeons passes a resolution "that some system of standardization of hospital equipment and hospital work should be developed."

1913 The American College of Surgeons (ACS) is incorporated in Illinois. It is formed from the Clinical Congress of Surgeons to recognize the distinction between those who are trained surgical specialists and those who are not. The "end result" system becomes a stated ACS objective.

1914 The American College of Surgeons (ACS) hires John G. Bowman as its first director. Bowman secures a $30,000 grant from the Carnegie Foundation that will lead to the formation of a hospital standardization program.

1915 The American College of Physicians (ACP) is founded.

1917 Editor John Hornsby of *Modern Healthcare* estimates that $1.445 billion is invested in hospital land and buildings.

Three hundred ACS fellows along with sixty leading hospital superintendents meet in Chicago for a three-day conference establishing the principle that knowledgeable professionals should assess hospital conditions and endeavor to achieve consensus among themselves on standards that will have the greatest effect on improving patient care. This principle will become fundamental to hospital standardization and later to hospital accreditation.

1918 The Codman Hospital closes. Codman publishes his record of the hospital in book, *A Study in Hospital Efficiency: As Demonstrated by the Case Report of the First Five Years of a Private Hospital*.

The American College of Surgeons (ACS) initiates a hospital standardization program, surveying 100-bed hospitals to determine a "minimum standard" of care. Only 89 of 692 hospitals surveyed meet the requirements.

1922 With the minimum standard in place, the American College of Surgeons' (ACS) survey program expands to include medium-size hospitals (those with 50 to 99 beds).

1924 Franklin Martin becomes director of the American College of Surgeons (ACS).

1926 The American College of Surgeons (ACS) publishes its first *Manual of Hospital Standardization*. The manual consists of 18 pages.

1940 Ernest A. Codman dies.

1941 The American College of Surgeons' (ACS) hospital standardization program has an operating budget of $44,000.

1946 The federal government places great reliance on the American College of Surgeons' (ACS) hospital certification program when it enacts legislation (the Hill-Burton Act) to fund hospital construction around the country.

1949 The American College of Surgeons' (ACS) hospital standardization program's budget has grown to $68,500.

1950 The American College of Surgeons (ACS) names Paul R. Hawley director.

A total of 3,290 hospitals, representing half the hospitals in the United States, are on the American College of Surgeons' (ACS) hospital standardization program's approved list.

1951 The American College of Physicians (ACP), the American Hospital Association (AHA), the American Medical Association (AMA), and the Canadian Medical Association (CMA) join with the American College of Surgeons to create the Joint Commission on Accreditation of Hospitals, an independent, not-for-profit organization whose primary purpose is to provide voluntary accreditation. The Joint Commission is incorporated in Illinois in November.

The Joint Commission holds its first official meeting (an organizational meeting) at the Drake Hotel in Chicago on the morning of December 15.

1952 The Joint Commission begins operations with a professional staff of two and an annual budget of $70,000 in space at ACS headquarters, 660 North Rush Street in Chicago.

Edwin L. Crosby is approved as director of the Joint Commission in March at a salary of $25,000. He assumes the directorship in September.

1953 The Joint Commission publishes *Standards for Hospital Accreditation*.

1954 Edwin L. Crosby resigns from the Joint Commission to become executive director (chief executive) of the American Hospital Association (AHA). Kenneth B. Babcock succeeds Crosby as director in July.

A total of 2,900 hospitals have been accredited in the United States.

1956 The Stover Committee recommends that the Joint Commission discontinue the use of voluntary surveyors and instead employ and oversee surveyors directly. A subsequent American Hospital Association (AHA) task force reaches the same conclusion.

1958 The Joint Commission begins to include medical staff appointments as part of accreditation criteria.

The Canadian Medical Association resigns its representation on the Joint Commission board in December to form its own accrediting organization in Canada.

1960 The Kerr-Mills Act institutes a program through which states that choose to participate will reimburse accredited hospitals for care of indigent patients. Kerr-Mills demonstrates third-party payers are not only recognizing Joint Commission accreditation as an indicator of good patient care, but they are beginning to require it as a condition of reimbursement.

1961 The Joint Commission makes fire safety a major priority in accreditation as Babcock asserts, "No matter how excellent the medical care, a hospital that is a fire trap will not be accredited."

1962 A total of 3,947 hospitals are accredited by the Joint Commission.

The Joint Commission, which has accredited hospitals in six countries other than the United States, decides not to accredit any more foreign hospitals because of a shortage of personnel.

1964 On January 1, the Joint Commission begins charging for surveys.

The total number of accredited hospitals increases to 4,287.

In October, Kenneth B. Babcock resigns from the directorship, and Denver Vickers becomes acting director.

The Joint Commission moves into its own offices at 201 East Ohio Street.

1965 The regulatory role of the Joint Commission is greatly augmented by the passage of Medicare legislation, as hospitals accredited by the Joint Commission are "deemed" to be in compliance with most of the Medicare conditions of participation and thus able to receive government reimbursement.

John D. Porterfield III assumes the directorship on June 15.

The Joint Commission board is expanded to include two additional representatives with regular three-year terms, one from the American Association of Homes for the Aging and one from the American Nursing Home Association.

1966 The Joint Commission enters into a contract with the newly-formed Commission on Accreditation of Rehabilitation Facilities (CARF), which offers accreditation services to rehabilitation centers, sheltered workshops, and organized programs for the homebound.

The Joint Commission finds a new home in the Blair Building at 645 North Michigan Avenue.

1969 The Joint Commission establishes the Accreditation Council for Services for the Mentally Retarded and Other Developmentally Disabled Persons.

The Joint Commission has approximately 65 employees.

1970 The Joint Commission establishes the Accreditation Council for Psychiatric Facilities.

Registered nurses and hospital administrators join physicians in conducting accreditation surveys.

The Joint Commission board approves revised standards for accreditation that represent optimal achievable levels of quality, rather than minimal essential levels of quality.

1971 The Joint Commission establishes the Accreditation Council for Long Term Care.

The Joint Commission's *Accreditation Manual for Hospitals*, intended to help educate and prepare hospitals for the accreditation process, is published in a loose-leaf binder in April.

1972 The Joint Commission has 170 employees.

The Social Security Act is amended to require that the secretary of the U.S. Department of Health and Human Services (DHHS) validate Joint Commission findings. The law also requires the secretary to include an evaluation of the Joint Commission's accreditation process in the annual DHHS report to Congress.

The first issue of *Perspectives* is published.

1973 Sister Virginia Schwager, an American Hospital Association (AHA) representative and Catholic nun, becomes the first woman to serve on the board of the Joint Commission.

The Joint Commission moves its offices to the 22nd floor of the towering John Hancock building at 875 North Michigan Avenue.

The Bureau of Health Insurance in the Social Security Administration begins to sends out validation teams. The teams are strictly inspectional, heavily emphasizing physical plant, building codes, and fire safety.

1974 The Joint Commission begins publishing the *Quality Review Bulletin*, offering practical assistance on quality assurance activities and patient care evaluation techniques. It is designed to meet the needs of a variety of staff members in the field.

1975 The Joint Commission establishes its newest accreditation council — the Council for Ambulatory Health Care — to accredit facilities in the burgeoning field of non-hospital health services.

As a result of the Bureau of Health Insurance's validation teams, 105 hospitals have lost their "deemed status," two-thirds because of life safety issues. The Bureau of Health Insurance disregards the Joint Commission's objections to the conduct of the validation surveys and denies it any channel through which to appeal validation decisions. The Joint Commission hires consultants to help it preserve the link between Joint Commission accreditation and "deemed status."

1976 The Joint Commission celebrates its 25th anniversary with a formal dinner at Chez Paul in Chicago on December 17.

The Federal Trade Commission initiates a preliminary investigation of the Joint Commission for suspected antitrust violations. Charges are never filed.

The Joint Commission is named as a co-defendant in the *Wilk* case, which questions the fairness of hospital staffing policies. Charges against the Joint Commission are eventually dismissed.

1977   John Affeldt takes over the directorship from Porterfield in August.

1978   At a special meeting on October 28, the Joint Commission's board institutes a reorganization plan terminating the four accreditation councils, and establishing Professional and Technical Advisory Committees (PTACs) to provide professional and technical advice to each of the relevant programs. (In addition to the four programs that had accreditation councils, there would be a separate PTAC for the hospital program.)

1979   The American Dental Association (ADA) is added as a corporate member of the Joint Commission.

The U.S. General Accounting Office releases a report, two years in the making, which constitutes an endorsement of the Joint Commission.

1981   The Joint Commission receives another Kellogg Foundation grant to develop standards and a self-assessment for hospice programs to care for terminally ill patients and their families.

1982   William G. Mitchell, a Chicago lawyer and businessman who was president of Central Telephone and Utilities Corporation, becomes the first public member of the board.

The two-year accreditation cycle is replaced by a three-year cycle for all programs except long-term care. (The cycle is changed to three years for long-term care in 1983.)

The hospice accreditation program is approved by the board in August and begins operation the following year. (It is folded into the home care program in 1990.)

1984   The Joint Commission's annual operating budget is $22 million. It has 411 employees, 243 in Chicago and another 168 surveyors in the field.

1985   The Joint Commission comes under attack for trying to keep some information gained during the survey process confidential, leading to contempt charges for Affeldt. An Illinois Supreme Court rules that the Illinois shield law protects the Joint Commission's actions and clears Affeldt. Subsequent court rulings in Florida, New York, and Texas come to the same conclusion.

The International Society for Quality Assurance (ISQA), a Swedish organization, gives the Joint Commission a seat on its board.

1986   John Affeldt retires and Dennis O'Leary assumes the directorship in April.

Affeldt and O'Leary present an issue paper to the board entitled, "An Agenda for Change." This project is intended to refine or delete many organizational structures and function standards that exist in Joint Commission standards manuals, placing a stricter focus on standards that are demonstrably important to the provision of quality care.

Quality Healthcare Resources is formed as a not-for-profit consulting subsidiary of the Joint Commission.

1987   Task forces are established to formulate clinical indicators in two areas of hospital care — obstetrics and anesthesia.

Yet another task force on organization and management indicators adopts principles of continuous quality improvement (CQI). This will soon become fundamental to the revision of all standards.

The Joint Commission changes its name from the Joint Commission on Accreditation of Hospitals to the Joint Commission on Accreditation of Healthcare Organizations.

The Joint Commission has accredited 5,400 hospitals and more than 3,000 non-hospital organizations.

The board authorizes initiation of home care accreditation surveys, using a comprehensive set of new standards to address the entire spectrum of home care services.

1988   The Joint Commission begins to conduct opinion surveys of hospital CEOs to establish a baseline for its customers' level of satisfaction.

The board approves the addition of two more seats for public members, raising board membership to 24. The new members join the board in 1990.

Development of the Indicator Measurement System (IMSystem) as an indicator-based performance monitoring system gets underway.

The Joint Commission begins accreditation of home care organizations.

1989   The Joint Commission quietly initiates a managed care accreditation program.

1990   The Joint Commission moves to new offices outside Chicago in Oakbrook Terrace on April 10.

A follow-up survey of hospital CEOs shows a marked improvement in how they viewed Joint Commission performance over the prior years.

The managed care program is terminated in May.

1992   The *Accreditation Manual for Hospitals* begins the multiyear transition to standards that emphasize performance improvement concepts.

A new standard is added requiring that all hospitals have a policy prohibiting smoking.

The board approves expansion to 28 seats, adding three more public representatives and one at-large representative of the nurse profession. The at-large nursing seat and one public member seat are filled the following year, with the remaining public seats being filled in 1994.

1993   The Joint Commission has accredited more than 3,000 home care organizations.

Random, unannounced surveys of 5 percent of accredited organizations begin.

The federal government announces that home health agencies accredited by the Joint Commission after an unannounced survey will be "deemed" to meet the Medicare Conditions of Participation.

The *Accreditation Manual for Hospitals* is reorganized around important patient care and organization functions to shift the focus from standards that measure an organization's capability to perform to those that look at its actual performance.

1994   The Joint Commission launches an accreditation program for health care networks.

Health care spending in the United States has reached $1 trillion, representing 14 percent of gross domestic product.

The *1995 Accreditation Manual for Hospitals, 1995 Accreditation Manual for Home Care* and *1995 Accreditation Manual for Mental Health, Chemical Dependency, and Mental Retardation/Developmental Disabilities Services* are published, completing the transition for these programs to performance-focused standards organized around functions important to patient care.

At a press conference in December, the AHA publicly criticizes the Joint Commission. O'Leary responds to this crisis of confidence by developing an Action Plan to address AHA concerns.

1995 The Joint Commission's home care accreditation program is conducting more surveys on an annual basis than the hospital accreditation program.

The federal government recognizes Joint Commission laboratory accreditation services as meeting the requirements for Clinical Laboratory Improvement Amendments of 1988 (CLIA) certification.

For the first time, a public member serves as an officer of the board of commissioners.

The *1996 Accreditation Manual for Ambulatory Health Care, 1996 Accreditation Manual for Health Care Networks, 1996 Accreditation Manual for Long Term Care* and *1996 Accreditation Manual for Pathology and Clinical Laboratory Services* are published, completing the transition for all programs to performance-focused standards organized around functions important to patient care.

1996 The Joint Commission reprints Ernest Codman's book, *A Study in Hospital Efficiency*.

The Joint Commission begins to formulate specific policies on sentinel events, defined as serious undesirable occurrences that result in the loss of patient life, limb, or function.

Laptop technology is introduced for use during hospital surveys, and a preliminary report is introduced. As a result, analysis of hospital findings is shorter, with improved consistency between the exit conference and final report.

In the future, all other accreditation programs also will incorporate laptop technology.

The Health Care Financing Administration announces that ambulatory surgical centers accredited by the Joint Commission will be "deemed" as meeting or exceeding Medicare certification requirements.

1997 The Joint Commission launches the ambitious ORYX performance measurement initiative to integrate the use of outcomes and other performance measures into the accreditation process.

The Codman Award is given out for the first time. It recognizes outstanding achievement by health care organizations and individuals in the use of performance measurement to improve an organization's performance.

The Joint Commission collaborates with five universities in establishing the Academy for Healthcare Quality for post-graduate continuing education, but the academy is dissolved in 1999.

The Joint Commission establishes Joint Commission Resources (JCR). JCR then includes all domestic and international consulting and international accreditation activities.

The board decides on the concept of encouraging organizations to report sentinel events and the findings of their root cause analyses of those events.

Quality Check, a directory of Joint Commission accredited organizations and performance reports, becomes available on the Joint Commission Web site.

1999 The Office of Inspector General (OIG) issues an important report, *The External Review of Hospital Quality*.

The board approves a change in the wording of the mission statement: (new words are italicized) "The mission...is to *continuously* improve the *safety and* quality of care provided to the public."

The Institute of Medicine receives wide public attention for the report *To Err Is Human*, which details the numbers and frequency of medical errors in hospitals.

The Random Unannounced Survey Policy is revised, effective January 1, 2000. Organizations will receive no advance notice for random unannounced surveys.

The Joint Commission establishes a toll free hot line to encourage patients, their families, caregivers, and others to share concerns regarding quality of care issues at accredited health care organizations.

The Joint Commissions Resources board approves the first set of Joint Commission International Accreditation standards for hospitals.

2000 Joint Commission Resources (JCR) is expanded to include all Joint Commission education, publications, and continuous survey readiness (CSR) activities.

King-Bruwaert House becomes the first organization to be accredited under the Joint Commission's new assisted living accreditation program.

2001 The Joint Commission celebrates its 50th anniversary.